D1394897

MILLION PLUS ONE

David Hughes

ARTHUR H. STOCKWELL LTD
Torrs Park   Ilfracombe   Devon
Established 1898
www.ahstockwell.co.uk

British Library Cataloguing-in-Publication Data.
A catalogue record for this book is available
from the British Library.

By the same author:
Purple Jade
The Cloned Identity

ISBN 978-0-7223-4257-2
Printed in Great Britain by
Arthur H. Stockwell Ltd
Torrs Park   Ilfracombe
Devon

DAVID'S FRIENDS AND FAMILY

Sheila Heritage, teacher and very special friend of David.

Jennifer, David's former wife.

Gregory, David and Jennifer's oldest son.

Joshua, Gregory's son and David's first grandchild, born just before David's accident.

Bethany, Gregory's daughter and David's second grandchild.

Heidi, David and Jennifer's daughter, now a major in British Army.

Phillip, David and Jennifer's youngest son.

Terry, David's brother, died 1947, aged five.

Stewart Terrance, David's brother.

Peter Alfred, David's brother, died August 2011, aged sixty.

Paul Malcolm, David's brother, twin brother to Peter.

John Barry, David's youngest brother.

John Ogg, head of science, died December 2006.

John Essam, CDT technician, died 2006.

Mrs Roberts, head teacher at the school where David worked.

Roly, head of the sixth form at the school.

Mal Bell, head of the CDT department at the school.

Kathy Kember, teacher, the only person who has ever given David flowers (yellow roses).

Dr Richard Garton, BDS, dentist at Castle Circus Health Centre.

Mr N. Sudhakar, FRCS, consultant neurosurgeon.

Malcolm Grant, coach at Brixham Archery Club.

INTRODUCTION BY SHEILA HERITAGE

DEATH ROW

This is a unique true story simply because David sustained a head injury so severe that he was not expected to survive; if he did, it was thought that he would be reduced to a vegetable state in a wheelchair. The fact that he not only survived but recovered to a level where he is able to write a book so concise and detailed about his life is totally amazing.

David was called 'the amazing man' by doctors. He was called 'one in a million' by consultants. And he was called 'a blooming miracle' by many others.

At the school where David worked for eighteen years he was a very important person in many different ways. He was not just an IT expert; he was also extremely knowledgeable in many other fields, and as such was always available to be of help and give his advice. He assisted in the building improvements and helped to solve staff home-computer problems as well as life's problems in general. He always seemed to be in the building from early to late, and always had time for both staff and pupils. He was always fair and honest in his appraisal of persons, and he had the ability to make people feel important and not useless. He always seemed to be your best friend because he never expected or wanted anything in return.

So you can imagine the general feelings in September 2005 when the staff returned to work after the summer break and David was not there as usual to greet them and make them feel at home; instead they read my statement explaining that he was in hospital with little chance of survival. A very solemn mood descended into the staffroom and many tears were shed.

Because David was on a life-support machine and in a coma for a considerable time, and had no knowledge of what had happened or was happening to him, the first part of this book contains extracts from a diary I kept at the time.

On 4 August 2005 David, who lives on his own, fell in his garden while pruning a tree. It was later assumed that he had fallen from a height of ten feet and had fallen backwards. He may have had a stroke. He landed on the patio, and the right side of his head struck the end of a steel scaffold pole sticking out of the ground. He fractured his skull, causing serious damage to the brain.

His neighbour, who would normally have been away that week, was at home and luckily he noticed David lying on the ground. When he didn't respond to the neighbour's questions, the neighbour climbed over the fence and realised he was seriously injured. He immediately called for an ambulance and, as the house was so close to the hospital, paramedics were there in four minutes. Because of the seriousness of the injury, they were unable to stabilise David and called for additional help. It took the four paramedics some time to stabilise him and transport him to the A & E department.

On his arrival they found that he had a very low monitor output, and the hospital's experience of severe head injuries led them to believe he was destined to be a mortuary case.

Luckily, because he maintained a pulse, the doctors rang Derriford Hospital in Plymouth (a specialist hospital for head injuries) and they agreed to take him. It was decided not to use the air ambulance because the vibrations of the helicopter might be fatal; instead he was transferred by road ambulance and, despite the concerns, he arrived still with a pulse.

At Derriford Hospital he underwent brain surgery to remove a blood clot. There was extensive bruising and damage to the brain. David was heavily sedated and put on a life-support machine in the neurological intensive care unit. His family and friends were informed that the chance of David surviving was very remote, so they prepared themselves for the worst.

However, David remained in this condition. The doctors were concerned about his high temperature, which they thought indicated an infection under the bone flap where they had originally operated, and on 18 August he was again taken to theatre for another operation, this time to remove the flap of bone from his skull.

On 21 August they 'turned off' the sedation and we waited for him to come round. We were told that it would take some time because of the amount of drugs that had been pumped into him over the past weeks.

He was transferred to the Moorgate haemodialysis unit on 26 August, where he continued to cause concern because of his high temperature and chest infection. By Bank Holiday Monday (29 August) he was showing some response. His eyes were following movements and he seemed a little more alert. It was quite macabre. He lay perfectly still and looked so peaceful. Although his eyes moved, there was no other response.

CHAPTER ONE

SHEILA'S DIARY

Monday 29 August
David seemed much brighter this morning – definitely following people moving past with his eyes and moving his head a little! When I went back to see David in the afternoon he seemed very tired and was definitely not so alert. He reacted to Paul's voice. I stayed until about seven o'clock when Jennifer arrived with Phillip.

Tuesday 30 August
This morning David looked similar to yesterday, but sleeping lots and not quite so alert. The male nurse had just spruced him up a bit, so perhaps he had tired him out. I asked if he could sit him up so that he could see a bit more, and he did, but David still slept. They have deflated something in his trachea, which is making him work harder to breathe, but he seems to be coping with it. The nurse said that the line in his neck is infected and that they are not able to put a peripheral line in anywhere else, so they will be taking him into theatre again in order to put another line in – this time on the left. He could not be any more specific as to when they would be taking him to theatre – we just have to wait and see.

They were not able to put one in on the left of his neck for some reason, so they had to put in a 'tunnel line'. It starts from the chest, but where it goes from there I don't know. They took an X-ray soon after he came back from theatre and the surgeon who did it came quite soon after to see the X-ray so that he could check that the line was in the right place. After all the activity and yet another general anaesthetic he just slept through my afternoon/evening visit. When the nurse tried to reconnect his oxygen line he could not get the machine which heats the oxygen to work. He went to get another one, but he couldn't get that one working either and I didn't want to leave until it was sorted. The night nurse managed to get the first one working in the end, but Paul and I did not leave until going up to eight.

Wednesday 31 August
David seemed brighter again this morning, and when I squeezed his hand I felt a twitch – as if he was trying to squeeze back. He also showed pain when they moved his leg. He turned his head from side to side to look at people talking to him, but he gave no response. The physiotherapists sat him upright on the edge of the bed (supported) and he seemed to cope with it OK. They did say that maybe they would try to put him in a chair soon. They seemed pleased. Altogether things seemed more positive today.

Thursday 1 September
We could not get in to see David at first this morning. Paul said that the curtains were drawn when he arrived. I did not arrive until about eleven o'clock, and we waited for a while in the relative's quiet room. After a while I asked at the nurses' station why we were not able to see him. One of the nurses went to check and said that he was 'dirty', so we had to wait until he had had a bed change. The physios hadn't been in, so he had not been put in a chair. He was not so alert this morning – slept a lot. Jennifer and Phillip were going to see him this afternoon, so I said I would be there at about five o'clock. It was hard in our visiting because we were all talking and relating to one another, but David was not involved. It wasn't that we were ignoring him, but it seemed as though he was there only in body. Maybe talking also made us feel secure, and perhaps somehow he was able to hear our voices and gain some support from our presence.

The central line which had been inserted in his neck was infected, and on 30 August he was taken to theatre so that they could insert another line. This morning we were informed that as well as the chest infection David now probably has MRSA.

Paul was waiting for me when I arrived later, and he said that he had some bad news. They had been told that David had MRSA. More drugs, more fighting, more worries! Jennifer said that David had been smiling for them and 'laughing' at something Phillip had said – but by the time I got there he was just sleeping and coughing. I shed quite a lot of tears – I feel at low ebb tonight. How much longer can he keep on fighting?

Friday 2 September
We arrived at the hospital at about 10.30 a.m. Peter and Paul were there, but we had to wait for a while before we could visit. It was their birthday and David gave them the best present ever: during the course of the day he became more and more aware and responsive. It seemed incredible. After the almost imagined twitches came a smile on request, a slight squeeze of the hand and a very definite smile of recognition. Everybody shed tears today. The shock of MRSA seems to have been dimmed by the improvement today. He still has a serious chest infection, and he still cannot talk or move other than a nod of the head, a smile and some finger movement; he still has MRSA, but he recognises us all; he can remember some things and *he is back*. I packed up the caravan and came home, but I feel as though he has turned a corner. I floated home.

Saturday 3 September
Jennifer was visiting in the afternoon, so I drove down to Derriford just after 9.30 a.m. Peter, Paul and I had to wait before we could go in to visit, but yesterday's improvements were not just a fluke – today there has been even more movement and he is even more responsive. I stayed with him while the physio worked with him. He obviously still has trouble with the chest infection as he is unable to take deep breaths, but the physio did some work to help to loosen the mucus in his lungs. Then she worked on his limbs. He can flex his fingers, but has a problem with the third finger of the left hand – it isn't as mobile as the others. Then she got him to wiggle his toes and helped him to move his arms and legs. There was definitely a flicker of movement in his muscles as he was trying to move for himself. She said it would be good for his chest if he were to sit up

more, and they said they would try to put him in a chair for a while. When morning visiting was over we left, and Peter and I went to the pub! When we went back they were still trying to get him into the chair, but soon afterwards we were able to go in and see him sitting up and watching what was going on. Heidi and Jennifer arrived soon after that, so I came home. He was sitting up for about an hour before they put him back into bed exhausted!

Sunday 4 September

Jennifer visited this morning with Heidi. Peter and John were also there. I met Peter and John at the Jack Rabbit at 1.30 p.m. and we went back to visit at 2.30. Gregory turned up at about three o'clock. David seemed to be quite tired today, and, although he is still progressing, he seemed a little down compared with yesterday. He still squeezes my hand and responds to requests to wiggle his toes, etc., but he doesn't seem quite as happy as yesterday. The timing of things like his splints and the nebuliser seem a bit haphazard, and some of his coughs had specks of blood in them. The nurse, Andy, said that the suction sometimes produces trauma, which I understand to mean that when the tube goes down the throat it can scratch. The blood is the colour I would expect from a scratch.

Monday 5 September

Today was my first day back at school, but a non-pupil day. I put up the statement in the staffroom about David so that I don't have to repeat myself and everyone is very concerned. Mrs Roberts was almost in tears when I told her that David had come round and that he is doing well – she was so pleased and relieved. I went to see him after school, leaving school a little early to miss the traffic. He has made more progress today. They have tried a swallow test on him: he was given a couple of spoonfuls of chocolate custard and he managed to swallow most of it successfully. They have fitted a speech valve in his throat, and he managed a faint "Hello." He was very positive tonight – constantly moving his limbs in order to try to get everything working again. He can move his legs quite a lot now. He seems to remember work and things that happened before his fall, but he seems very vague about events afterwards. The nurse suggested an audio book might keep him interested; there is nothing much he can do except lie in bed.

Tuesday 6 September

I went to the library at lunchtime to find an audio book. They are nearly all on cassette, so I also went to Argos to try to buy a mains personal tape player. I have not been very successful as the one I bought has a socket for mains supply, but there is no supply. Instead I took my tape player from school. I left school at about 3.20 because I was not teaching the last lesson. Jennifer was going to see him this evening, but I wanted to see him as well. I had to stop for petrol, but I arrived on the ward about 4.45.

What a shock – he can speak! The trachea tube has been replaced with a narrower one. His voice is very quiet, but he is able to communicate with us. He asked for a drink and there was a cup with a straw by his bed, so I let him have some. Later a nurse came round and I told her, and she said he was 'nil by mouth'. How are we expected to know? Anyway, he managed. He is very confused and just kept repeating that it was 'very odd'. He starts to say something, but cannot always finish – it is very hard work for him. He also kept saying that he wants to go home. I asked him if he could remember where he was, and he knew he was in Plymouth but didn't know the name of the hospital. He was very worried about Phillip – he said he had to take him somewhere. I think he was due to take Phillip to the airport for his holiday, but Phillip cancelled his holiday when David had the fall. He was also concerned about painting Phillip's room. I kept telling him that Phillip would be in to see him very soon – he was due to be there at 6.45. Although it was very good to see him talking – a big step forward – I found the visit very upsetting. He seems so fragile, so confused. It is very frightening for him – and me.

Wednesday 7 September

Today I had some good news and some disappointing news about David. The good news is that he is now in Torbay rather than Plymouth; the disappointing news is that I didn't find out until I was on the ward in Plymouth! They said they tried to phone, but no one picked up the phone – presumably they didn't like to leave a message on the answerphone. I had a wasted journey to Derriford and back, but never mind.

They seem very nice on the ward in Torbay. Talk about a major shock! He is in the stroke unit – George Earl Ward. He is in a room on his own at the moment because of the MRSA.

When I walked into the room he was on his side, and he looked up at me and reacted like nothing had happened. His words were "Hello. Been to Plymouth. Banged my head. Just waiting for the doctor, then you can take me home."

To say I was flabbergasted is an understatement. I have just spent weeks going practically nonstop to Plymouth to visit him while he lay dormant, never knowing if he would survive, having little or no response to my attempts at conversation, and now there he was behaving as if nothing had happened. I told him I didn't think he was ready to go home just yet.

Because of the MRSA he will be swabbed again on Friday, and if he is clear, he will go on to the ward with others – which the sister said will be better for him. He is still confused, but, considering the day he must have had with the journey in the ambulance from Plymouth and all the new people and surroundings to get used to, he seems very well. He seemed very pleased to see me – a familiar face when everything around him had changed. His room is nice with a window from which he can see the moors. The sky was very pretty this evening in the setting sun. They gave me lots of leaflets to look at, and I went through some of them with him. They all seem very honest but positive – they say the main goal is to get people back to their own home, etc. David still keeps saying he wants to go home; and I keep telling him we all want him to be back in his own home as soon as possible, but he must stay in hospital until he is a bit stronger. I told him about John Essam being in the same ward when he had his stroke and how he is now back at home and driving again. By the time I was due to go home he seemed quite calm and sleepy. I think he should sleep well tonight.

Thursday 8 September
I left school promptly at the end of the day and was in the ward by just after four o'clock. I stayed with David for a couple of hours. He seemed quite down today. He just keeps saying that he wants to go home. He had pulled the tube from his nose earlier in the day and he had missed out on a litre of Jevity (the liquid feed), so he was hungry. He said no one had been in to him, but I am sure that the physios, etc. had been in. He is still 'nil by mouth' apart from a couple of spoons of custard every now and again until his swallow has improved. The nurse said they may remove the trachea tube soon. The ward sister came in and cleaned around the line in his chest. The dressing had not been changed since the 5th and it was clear that at some time there had been some bleeding – the blood had soaked through the dressing. She cleaned it up and replaced the dressing with a clear one so that you could see the line without disturbing the dressing. He was still only wearing a hospital gown, and it looked like the one I saw them put on him yesterday.

Friday 9 September
I went to the hospital at about 3.30 p.m. because I was not teaching during the last period. David was in a chair by the side of his bed, and he was wearing a shirt and shorts. There was a dressing over his throat, and it looks as though they have removed the tube (although I did not speak to anyone to confirm this). He seemed much more with it and, although he still keeps saying that he wants to go home, he participated in and initiated some conversation. He was talking about his Magnum and about cycling. A nurse came into the room to put him back into bed – there is a hoist built into the ceiling. She is from Poland and David seemed to take a shine to her. However, he did start saying some rubbish about cycling in Poland. I don't know how long he had been in the chair, but he seemed more comfortable lying flat in bed for a while. Peter, Paul and Denise came about five o'clock and he seemed very pleased to see them. He knew who they were and again initiated conversation about topics associated with Paul and Denise – a holiday in Turkey, horses . . . He is still not allowed to eat and is still complaining of being hungry. There were a couple of photos of

Joshua with his cards; I commented that I could see Gregory in his face, and David said he could also see Louise. Sometimes he is quite lucid; at other times he is confused. At times he also tries to make jokes, although I am not sure that everyone else understands. He still cannot always finish his sentences.

Jennifer and Heidi arrived about six o'clock, so I left. Peter had arranged for the four of us to go out for a meal, and I had booked a table at the Ocean Drive on the corner of Walnut Road – it was a good evening.

Saturday 10 September
Jennifer and Heidi wanted to go to see David early in the afternoon, so I went about four o'clock. Peter, Paul and Denise were there and David was in bed. Peter said David had been quite down when they arrived and just wanted to go home. I found out from the nurse later that he had had another bowel movement, and when I spoke to Jenny I realised that they may have been there at the time. If that was the case, it explains why he was so distressed – but I may be wrong. Anyway, he seemed in quite good spirits when I arrived, and he joined in with some of the conversation – although some of it was fantasy. He kept complaining that he was cold and they brought him an extra blanket. His brothers left about five.

The Filipino nurse was looking after him today. I had told her that he preferred ice cream to custard, and she brought in a little tub. I was able to give him a couple of spoons – most of which he swallowed. He had slithered down the bed and was starting to cough more. The coloured nurse adjusted the bed so that he was more upright, which stopped the coughing. He was very tired after all his visitors today and I suggested that he have a little nap – I told him I would stay with him – so he slept while I held his hand. About 7.30 they came in to settle him down for the night, so I left.

Sunday 11 September
Jennifer went in early in the afternoon, so I said I would be in later. I had some marking to do, so I arrived just before five o'clock. David was a bit fed up again, and the nurse said he had been asking for me. He is still desperate to go home. I explained again that he

would not be able to go home until he was clear of the chest infection, and was able to eat properly and walk on his own. Each day he seems a little stronger. He moves his legs much more, and he can lift his arms as well as his hands. Because it is Sunday there were no physios in, and when nothing is happening he gets bored, frustrated and depressed. He still keeps sliding down the bed.

I tried to get him to sit up a bit more by himself because it helps his breathing, but when he pushed against the end of the bed it just came off. He was able to grasp the sides of the bed and lift himself up a bit, so his arms are getting stronger.

I gave him some more ice cream, but the nurse said he hadn't had enough. I am a little confused because it says he should have only three teaspoons at a time, which is what he had. But she said he didn't want it earlier in the day. I need to be able to talk to the speech therapists – the nurses only do as they are told!

One of the ancillary staff spoke to me this afternoon – it turned out to be Sasha from school. She had been working at the hospital in her summer break from university; unfortunately it is her last day today or she would have gone in to talk to David tomorrow. I really think he needs more stimulation. When I spoke to Peter tonight he suggested that I take in a newspaper tomorrow. I will take something easy like *The Sun* – I think he prefers *The Express* or *The Mail*, but *The Sun* will be easier to start with.

Jennifer had bought him some new tracksuit bottoms; but they looked a bit small to me, so I asked him where his were at home. He said they were in his wardrobe. When I left I called in at his house and looked, and they were where he said they would be. I will take them in tomorrow.

Monday 12 September
Not a good day! Nothing seems to be happening. I was told that he couldn't have ice cream, even though he had already been having it; I went home and made him some apple purée, but I was told he couldn't have that either. No one seems to have been with him much today and he was very depressed.

16

Tuesday 13 September

Peter phoned the hospital and told them what he thought of them, and I phoned and asked to make an appointment to speak to the speech therapist. She was waiting for me when I arrived, and we went into David's room to have a chat. I explained my concerns, and she went through a few things with us.

Wednesday 14 September

I left my mobile at school when I went home for lunch. When I got back there was a voicemail message from the hospital saying they were moving David to Newton Abbot. I phoned, but they could not give me a time when he was going. I wasn't teaching, so went straight over. David was very upset because they had told him they were moving him and had packed his things into carrier bags and then just left him. The ambulance men arrived soon after I did and took him straight away. I went back to work to shut down my computer, etc. and went straight over to Newton Abbot. I expected him to be still upset, but when I arrived he seemed quite happy. He was in a room of his own, with a wardrobe, TV, washbasin, commode and still some space. They had put up his cards and photos of Joshua and made him feel welcome.

Thursday 15 September

I went to see David after school, arriving about 4.15. There were lots of places to park. I went straight to his room. He seemed more lucid, but was a bit distressed. He had spent quite some time in the chair today, and it hurts his bottom to sit for any length of time.

Two speech therapists came in to assess him while I was there. They asked him to make various facial movements, etc., and then tried him on swallowing. He was given some thickened juice, which he managed reasonably well. They have said he can have thickened drinks and should be on ten spoonfuls of purée at mealtimes. He was a little concerned about his catheter, and later he wanted to go to the toilet. I called a nurse and they got him on to the commode. It must be very distressing for him to be so out of control when he has been such a private man. A few tears!

Generally, though, there has been still more progress today. I left about 5.30. Jennifer was due to go this evening.

Friday 16 September
I managed to get to the hospital for about four o'clock – the traffic was terrible. David was on the bed with a blanket over him, but he was still very cold. Every day there is more improvement and every day he becomes more talkative. Today we had some tears about his brother Terry. He became quite distressed. I stayed long after visiting hours had finished until he had cheered up a bit. Just before six o'clock the sister came in to start giving him his supper, etc., so I had to leave. Gregory and Heidi went to see him in the evening.

Saturday 17 September
Jennifer wanted to go out for the day, so I was able to visit this afternoon. When they opened the doors to let us in I went to his room, and as soon as David saw me he held out his arms and asked for a cuddle. My old David back again! He said he had missed me and was very glad to see me. He was on the bed with just a blanket over him and was very cold again, so I covered him with the rest of the bedclothes and asked for another blanket. It was more than an hour before he was warm again. I think what happens is that when he is put back in bed he is covered with a blanket for the sake of modesty, and he doesn't realise he is getting chilly until he is really cold. He is unable to cover himself up with blankets, so he just gets colder and colder.

I had gone into town during the morning to find him a lightweight sweatshirt with a full-length zip. He wouldn't wear a cardigan and I didn't want to get him something he had to put on over his head. I looked in every shop selling menswear. There was one in BHS, but it was knitted; and there were a couple in TK Maxx, but they had hoods. The best was one from Primark, so I bought it.

We talked all afternoon about all sorts, and he was able to think of most of the words he wanted. There was still a little talk of when he was in the police, which was a little disturbing, but other than that it was a good afternoon – the time flew by. He asked about his house, and I asked him what he had done with the set of keys that I had. He said "Ahh . . ." and proceeded to describe where he had put them.

He asked about his wallet. I think Peter said Jennifer was given it by the hospital, but I didn't tell him – it isn't my place. But I will tell Peter.

Once David was warm he started moving about more, using his arms and legs, and all too soon they rang the bell for visitors to leave. I went home via Sainsbury's because I had promised to cook a meal for John at David's house. I was expecting him about 8.30 because visiting finishes at 8 p.m., but Jennifer, Heidi and John arrived just after 7.30.

Sunday 18 September
Jennifer was due to pick up John at about 3 p.m., so I went visiting at two o'clock and left when they arrived. I visited again at seven o'clock and Mal turned up. David seemed quite pleased to see him.

Monday 19 September
I didn't think I would be able to see David today because Jennifer was going in the evening and I had a departmental meeting after school, but Caroline said I needn't go so I drove straight to Newton Abbot after school. Rhoda (the consultant therapist) came in to talk to us. I had arranged to meet her on Wednesday, but she asked if I was Miss Heritage and came in. She talked a lot to David about how he thought he was getting on and what he saw as his main problems. He told her it was his 'plumbing' which was a problem – it is probably due to the Jevity he is having pumped into him. He says that when they bring him his puréed food he tries to eat it, but he is already feeling very full. She told us the nutritionist comes in on Wednesday and maybe they would change his feeding regime to eating and then being topped up with Jevity. At the moment he is being asked to eat his dinner while the pump is running. She also said it may be possible to take him out for an hour or so at the weekend, which would be marvellous. She was very nice, and everything seemed positive. I asked her if she could confirm whether or not he has a urine infection, so she looked through his

notes and said that he was indeed on antibiotics for a urine infection – probably caused by the catheter. She said the catheter would not be removed until he was rid of the infection. When his waterworks and bowels are sorted and he has his feeding tube removed he can think about returning home.

Tuesday 20 September
When I arrived this afternoon David was talking to one of the speech therapists. She was making him 'jump through verbal hoops' – finding things in a picture, reading instructions and following them and describing what he saw in a picture. He did everything perfectly, and she said it was the best description of the picture she had heard. He is able to use a rich vocabulary and, although he still occasionally stumbles over a word, his language skills are about back to normal. He had had quite a busy day with the occupational therapist – Steve. He had to give himself a strip wash at the sink this morning, which seemed OK, but he is having some difficulty cleaning his teeth – his grip is not quite right (but it is improving) and his arm still shakes. He was not comfortable combing his hair because of the soft spot, so I will look for a soft brush for him. Kathy Kember had sent in some roses for him – yellow – and he seemed quite pleased. He's still improving. It's hard to get a word in sometimes – he is such a chatterbox.

Wednesday 21 September
I checked with Liz to see if it was OK to visit David this afternoon as I had no timetabled lessons, and she said yes so I was able to be with him from about 2.20. He was on the bed, dozing. He was in quite good spirits. He had washed himself again and said that he found the teeth-cleaning better today. He had spent some time with the occupational therapist again today, but he had not done any more walking. He has decided he does not feel ready to go on a home visit yet, but maybe he would like to be pushed around the hospital grounds for a little at the weekend. He wants to spend some time talking to Peter. He said he thinks that the idea of living in France may be too much for him, but he may downsize. He seems not to want all the hassle; he wants more peace. He said he

realises he is no longer a 100-mile-an-hour man. I reminded him about the day he responded to commands for the first time: it was on Peter and Paul's birthday and he poked his tongue out for them. I told him that they said it was the best present they could ever have had and that they both shed a tear. It made him cry. I wanted to make him happy, but it had upset him. I was trying to show him just how much progress he had made. I had taken in a couple of brushes for him, but they are still a bit too hard; he thinks he has some softer ones at home in cupboards or drawers in the hall, so I will look tomorrow.

The ward manager came in with some paperwork for us to fill in about David's background – almost the same as I filled in at Torbay, but the first one seems to have gone missing. Rhoda (the department manager) came in to see us and David told her he did not really think he was ready to go out. He said he knew he would need to be in hospital for another couple of weeks or so and he was OK with that – he doesn't want to rush things. I asked about the MRSA and she said that, even if he still had it when the time came for him to be discharged, it would not prevent him from being allowed to go home. It seems now that the wound in his neck where the trachea tube was is infected. They swabbed him again today, but we will have to wait for the results. We had quite a long chat about my girls' weddings/husbands and about his feelings.

Thursday 22 September
David was not feeling so good today. He had spoken to a doctor during the day and showed him his finger. The doctor said it should be X-rayed and they came to take him down the corridor while I was there. David was quite pleased to see some of the world outside his room. Between my leaving after the end of afternoon visiting and coming back for evening visiting the doctor had looked at the X-rays and said that the finger was dislocated. He tried to put it back, but was unable to do so. He said David should go to the fracture clinic at Torbay Hospital, and that has been arranged for tomorrow sometime. I don't know if the dietician has been in to see him or if she has just responded to Rhoda's request to change his feeding regime, but I think they are cutting back on his liquid

feed. I don't know the details, but I will ask as soon as the opportunity arises.

Friday 23 September
Jennifer phoned at 7.30 this morning to say she would be visiting David this afternoon and then she would be going away for a few days and would be back to visit him on Thursday evening.

I left school about three o'clock and phoned the hospital to see if David was back from the fracture clinic at Torbay. He wasn't and they suggested I phone later. I tried again about 3.45 and Sister Ann said the nurse that accompanied him had just phoned. She and David were waiting for patient transport and would not be back until at least five o'clock; he was in A & E and had not had anything to eat or drink all day. I grabbed a tin of custard from the cupboard, a tin-opener and a spoon and went to find him. He was in reasonable spirits under the circumstances, as was Mary – the nurse. He had been taken to the fracture clinic by ambulance, but without an appointment, as I understand, so he had to wait to be seen. The doctor gave him a couple of shots of local anaesthetic and tried to manipulate the dislocated finger back into place, but, because it had been out for so long, he was unable to do anything with it. So he strapped it, and then came the wait for transport back to Newton Abbot. He had been lying on a trolley all day as well. Mary organised some water to flush out his NG tube, and then I was able to give him some custard – and still we waited. One of the nurses on duty and I persuaded Mary to go and have a cup of coffee. Her shift was supposed to have finished at 4.30! Someone finally arrived to collect a patient for Brixham, but it seemed that there was no one in the department waiting for Brixham – just David and another lady, also on a trolley. They said they could only take one trolley and one chair and asked if David would be all right to travel in a chair. They checked with Mary and transferred him to a wheelchair. They finally left just before 6.30.

Peter, Paul and Denise are coming this weekend and were due to arrive about five o'clock, so I went to David's house to tell them what had happened. They went over to see him, and I went home to feed the dog and have a shower before going over. John Ogg had decided to visit (ignoring my request to consult with me so that too many people wouldn't arrive at once). David was sitting in a chair and they had given him some purée for his dinner. By the look of the empty plate, he must have been quite hungry! He was bothered by his eye, which seemed sore, and he kept rubbing it. He was also very tired and asked me to call the nurse so that he could go back to bed. We left about 7.45. I had booked a table at the Ocean Drive again – a good night.

Saturday 24 September
I made Paul a lemon meringue pie in the morning while Peter, Paul and Denise did some jobs at David's house. Peter changed the locks, Paul painted the railings and Denise tidied up his front garden. David was in bed for afternoon visiting – we all took it in turns so that there would not be too many people round his bed at once. Peter took in some flowers for the sister for her birthday and some chocolates for the nurses. When I visited in the evening David said how much he had enjoyed his afternoon.

Sunday 25 September
I asked David if he would like me to try to find a wheelchair so that I could take him for some fresh air, but he didn't want me to. He tried to explain why he didn't want to go out, and I think it was because it would be too overwhelming. We talked a lot and the time passed very pleasantly. It seems very quiet at weekends – there are no physios or occupational therapists in and not a lot seems to happen. They were very short-staffed today, and David said he was left in his bed until about 11.30. One of the nurses said they had had quite a number of new patients in and the ward was full. Mal turned up during evening visiting.

Monday 26 September
David was not in his room when I arrived this afternoon. I went to the nurses' station and was told that he was in the gym with the physio. He was sitting on the edge of a bench and Mark was asking him to reach to each side in turn to test him with his balance. David was getting tired. He walked back to his room and got into bed. He

told me that he had seen the occupational therapist earlier in the day and he asked me to bring in a laptop to show the occupational therapist that he could use the keyboard. I took it in for evening visiting and gave him the password, etc. They had found him some squash, which he seems to like the taste of, so I bought him some more and took that in too. He was in very good spirits today.

Tuesday 27 September
When I got to the hospital this afternoon David's bed hadn't been slept in and he wasn't in his room! I remembered that he was due to see the physiotherapist, so I went into the gym to see if I could find him there. He was standing unaided at a table taking pegs off nails! I suppose it was a task to test and improve manual dexterity. Anyway, he was able to do it all without any problem. Mark, the physio, said he needed to practise more walking, and they went up and down the corridor. David seems quite steady on his feet when he is going in a straight line – he walks unaided, but he has to concentrate and he is apt to lose his balance when he tries to turn.

I followed him back to his room and he sat in the chair. He was quite tired, but in very good spirits. There have been two more milestones to enjoy today. Firstly he had his catheter removed – he said it made his eyes water when they took it out, but he seems to have managed using a bottle without any problems. The other milestone is that he has moved from purée to soft, moist food – more of a normal diet. He seems to have enjoyed his lunch.

Roly picked me up and came with me to visit this evening. He had offered to pick me up because he didn't know where the hospital was. He asked if he should bring the sports car and I said a definite yes. He arrived in his BMW Z3. It is lovely – a very low, sleek, metallic silver automatic.

When we got to David's room I had quite a shock. David was in a bad state. He was very upset. He said that one of the nurses gave him some medication which was like chalk – some white powder in water. Anyway, it was very difficult for him to drink and it made his throat hurt. He had had his soup, but he said he did not have any more dinner – they had brought him some ice cream although we had said he did not want anything sweet. Some tears!

I asked to speak to the nurse and spoke to someone called Ann. She could not shed any light on what had happened, but she assured me that according to his chart he hadn't had anything unusual – perhaps he had been given the medication orally when he was used to it being given through the tube. Anyway, Roly and I talked to him and he seemed a little brighter when we left.

Wednesday 28 September
I went to the hospital in the afternoon as we had an appointment with the team looking after David. When I arrived he was with Steve and the door was shut. They finished soon after I arrived and I was able to go in. He was in quite good spirits. He had been to Torbay Hospital in the morning about his finger, and they had decided to leave well alone for the time being. I was called into the 'team meeting' just after 3.30. There was Rhoda, the nurse in charge of the 'red' team, a physiotherapist and a lady from social services. The physio said they were pleased with his progress, as did the report from the speech therapist. We discussed the timing for a home assessment visit. I explained that Wednesday would be the best day for me because of work commitments, etc., although it is not so good for them. It may be next Wednesday! Because of the MRSA I may have to take him in my car, which wouldn't be a problem. At least we have something to look forward to.

The nutritionist also came in to see David, and she recommended that he comes off the Jevity and relies on his meals. They are keeping the tube in his nose for now in case he becomes dehydrated. I came home and made him a tiny fish pie and took it back for evening visiting. Bless him – he had eaten tomato soup and macaroni cheese for his dinner, but still managed to eat my fish pie!

CHAPTER TWO

DAVID'S RECOLLECTION

My first real recollection was at Torbay Hospital. What made things so difficult for me was that I was never told exactly what had happened to me. All the time I was in hospital I was never told by either the medical staff or family and friends what had happened. In my mind I had just bumped my head, and because I was alive and, it seemed to me, well I could not understand why I was being treated in the way I was. In some ways I felt I was being punished and kept in hospital because of the problems I had caused. It became very important to me that I could get home and resume my normal life.

While at Torbay Hospital I was visited by Steve. He was the physio from Newton Abbot Hospital. He came in and looked at me and introduced himself, and said he was visiting Torbay Hospital. At that point I had worked out that the reason my arms and hands didn't work was because of the bang on my head, and I thought I just needed some physio to make them work again. I seemed to have discounted the mass of tubing coming out of me and the fact my legs, etc. didn't work. I just said to him I was waiting for the doctors to give me the OK to go home. He then said he would take me down to the gym to see how I was and left the room.

I thought I would give him a game of basketball just to show him there was nothing wrong with me.

After a few minutes he returned with a wheelchair and a couple of nurses. I thought that was just Health & Safety again, so I was not bothered. They got me in the chair and off we went. I was feeling quite happy until we went into the gym – well, the gym was just an empty ward which had a few very basic pieces of apparatus, so I was immediately disappointed. They got me out of the chair and sat me on a bed. Steve then attached a harness round my body and winched the apparatus up so that I was standing there. He asked me how I felt. I replied that I was fine. He looked at me and I smiled back, thinking, 'Right – I can go home now.' He then released the support and I just collapsed back on to the bed. A big shock for me!

I looked at him in total disbelief and said, "My God! My legs collapsed. What the hell have they done to me?"

At that moment I was totally convinced that the hospital had damaged my legs and it was their fault they didn't work properly. If someone had explained that I had been in hospital for a long time and, having no movement, all my muscles had wasted away until half my bodyweight had disappeared, then I might have been expecting what happened!

I was taken back to my bed, totally disillusioned – but not for long. Steve explained that he would arrange for me to be transferred to his hospital so he could sort me out; and from that moment I was sure he would have proper facilities and, because of my capabilities, it would just take a couple of days before I could go home.

It took, because of a problem with transport, a whole day before I arrived at Newton Abbot Hospital. I cheered up when I was taken past the ward and I was given my own room again. I thought that was because I would be there for only a couple of days. The staff were very good. They seemed to be pleased to see me, and they settled me in and kept popping in and out as they changed shift.

On the second day a lady appeared. She introduced herself and seemed to be in charge. I noticed she had a big thick folder, so I worked out that she was going round all the patients. Then she started telling me I had quite a large injury and it would take a while for me to recover. It seemed to me as though she was on another planet or had got me mixed up with someone else. I was sure there was nothing wrong with me that a couple of days couldn't sort out.

After she left I had a bit of a wobble. She had implied that I might be a vegetable in a wheelchair for the rest of my life, but that I could not accept. I became very agitated and tried to get out of the bed and go home, but I could not get over the sides (which were up). It took a while for me to stabilise, and I decided I would have to prove them wrong and me right.

The weeks I spent at Newton Abbot were OK in some ways. I was well looked after, although it seemed to me that most of what they did was based on the assumption that all the patients were the same.

Some of the staff would come and sit for a chat. They told me I was their best patient for looking after as a lot of the others were stroke victims and were always complaining about something. I had my mind set up that I had to be a model patient and convince the hospital that I was OK. I realised that the fact I lived on my own was an issue for some reason, but it seemed silly to me. Later on I realised that the hospital staff were all working for my best interest and they were far more aware of my condition than I was – or than I was able to accept. One problem I found was that they were not able to accept that I was not anything like the 'normal' patient. They weren't dealing with a difficult person, but with a totally different person to the norm, and they found it far more difficult to relate to me than I did to them.

One example: I was lying on my bed when a very nice lady came in with her folder (persons appearing with a folder was the norm). She spent a few minutes explaining that she was the speech therapist and she had come to help me learn how to communicate. She kept repeating everything. She said everything several times, very clearly. I was quite bemused and never said a word back. I was quite enjoying how she was performing and I realised she basically did not have a clue about me. Then she explained that she was going to say a sentence to me and I should see how much I could understand and repeat any words I could remember. I just looked at her.

She then said very clearly and concisely, "The cat sat on the mat."

I looked at her, showing no emotion, so she repeated it again. I rolled over in my bed and she panicked. She thought I was having a seizure and was about to fall out of bed.

She grabbed hold of me and said, "Mr Hughes, are you all right? Do you want a nurse – a doctor?"

I looked at her and said, "I can't see it."

She said, "What, Mr Hughes? What can't you see?"

I replied, "The cat you said sat on the mat. I didn't even see it come in."

She looked quite startled and said, "You heard and understood what I said!"

"Yes, but I would sooner talk about engineering, computer networks, boat design and building, etc., etc."

She looked totally gobsmacked and quickly looked through her folder. She looked at me, but I could tell from her face that she wasn't going to take me at face value. I thought it was because she was confused by my reaction, but much later I found out that people's reaction to my flippancy was often because they knew I wasn't so good as I thought and that I could expire at any time. A lot of the tests I was given were taken from American manuals and I complained that they were not relevant to me; I even offered to write the correct English version of the tests.

After a while at Newton Abbot I found myself getting bored during the day. I really needed to have more to do to cope with my lack of mobility. I started to become agitated at nothing happening. I felt I had completed all the tests and needed to go home or I would become a hospital vegetable.

I was taken home for an hour so that Steve and a colleague could make some assessment of my ability to look after myself in my home. My feelings were exactly what the hospital staff had told me to expect: it was a very emotional experience to enter my own home again. Since I was at Torbay Hospital there had been emotional storms as I thought I would never see it again. To be able to walk in and see my possessions was very special. I believed I had to comply with all the requirements and not be too flippant if I was to convince the hospital it would be safe for me to come home, so I did everything Steve asked me to do. I sat on the loo and stood up, sat down and stood up, went up and down the stairs, lay on my bed and got up, and went out into the garden, which I found particularly upsetting. My family had told me where I had been found, but I couldn't remember anything of the accident. Then I made a cup of tea and sat down to drink it. I realised later that this too was a test to see how safe I was. I listened to Steve and agreed with his suggestion that grab handles should be fitted in appropriate places.

We also discussed the danger of my falling down the stairs. In 2009 I did fall down the stairs. It was my fault – not concentrating. I smacked the right side of my head against the wall with quite a bang and hit the floor and lay still, expecting to expire at any moment. I was not able to reach any phone for help, and I was blocking the front door so no one would have been able to enter. After about thirty minutes I crawled into the front room and managed to climb into a chair and take stock. I believe I survived because my head hit the flat wall rather than a projection of some kind. I have now arranged things so that if the front door is blocked, persons can gain access through the back door; I also try to carry my mobile phone and keep it operational.

Another anxious moment was when I locked myself in the porch. I had had a new outer door and frosted window fitted a few months before so nobody could see in and I couldn't see out. I tried to call for help on the mobile, but none of the contact numbers I had were available. I tried banging on the window, but was unable to attract attention; so I put my umbrella out through the letter box and waggled it about. Some time later my opposite neighbour, Jo, came to my rescue. She had noticed the umbrella earlier, but thought I was painting. I was able to describe where my spare key was and she found it and unlocked my prison. I had been there for some three hours and was in a distressed state for quite a while, so she made a cup of tea and sat with me until I stabilised. Yes, I had thought about calling the fire brigade or police, but I was worried that they might call for an ambulance and I would be back in hospital and social would be told I was not looking after myself. The possibility of being put into care was a big worry for me for a very long time.

After my hour home trial I was allowed home for a weekend, and that weekend my brothers had arranged to stay at my house and visit me in the hospital. My friend Sheila, who had brought me home and was keeping an eye on me, had not told them I would be home, so when they arrived on the Saturday they did not expect me to be there. This was quite an emotional meeting for us.

On the Saturday evening we had a Chinese takeaway meal, which was the first time I had sat at a table and had real food since my accident. But I became tired very quickly as I was not used to so much talking and being with so many persons at once. Being looked after in my own home was a totally new experience. I felt worn out, so I went to bed early, but I found it difficult to sleep. I could still vaguely hear, in a sort of blur, the conversations going on downstairs.

On Sunday afternoon I returned to hospital as required. I was convinced that I should be allowed to go home and I became agitated as the assessment day at the hospital arrived. I could not see any reason why I could not be discharged, but time dragged on. I said I was getting to the stage when I would discharge myself.

The day finally arrived – 15 October, a week before my birthday. I was driven home. The traffic was bad and it seemed to take for ever before I was indoors again.

My good friend Sheila had agreed to stay with me for a couple of days; then my brother Peter was coming for a week as I had a list of hospital appointments to attend.

During my first week at home I had many visits from persons and departments, checking up and giving me tests to evaluate my condition.

Being at home meant I was becoming so much more aware of the problems I had. In hospital they didn't matter in the same way. All my physical deficiencies now became apparent. I was unable to walk properly. My arms, my fingers, my body, my muscles – nothing was working as it should, and all the simple everyday things were a struggle. I found out much later that because my system had been shut down for so long a lot of simple everyday things had to be relearnt by my brain. The first time I was taken out in the front seat of a car, for example, I could see all that was happening around me, but my head could not cope with the sheer volume of data that was pouring in so quickly and I became totally confused and upset.

As my physical condition improved, my mental state did not improve at the same rate. I found I was able to do physical tasks, but I became confused on the mental side. The first time I tried to eat an apple I found I could not open my mouth wide enough. My jaw seemed locked, and that was probably because I had been fed so long through tubes. I had to retrain my jaw to get it to work again.

I want to thank the Dutch physio lady from Torbay Hospital who came to my home. The first time she took hold of my legs and arms I felt as though I was being pulled apart. It was quite a shock to the system, but it showed me just how far I was away from being well again. On the following visits she had me outside and walking, and she made it possible for me to walk from my home down the dreaded hill. I was concerned that I might fall backwards and not be able to protect my head. She took me to the bus stop and showed me how to get on and off the buses safely. She also gave me diagrams of exercises I should undertake. Later I was able to visit her at the hospital so that she could evaluate my progress.

During my first week at home my brother took me to the supermarket as I wanted to get the food I used to like before my accident. I managed to cook a simple meal myself as before.

When we sat down and ate it I was disappointed because of the taste and I apologised to him for messing up, but he said it tasted nice and there was nothing wrong. At the time I thought he was being kind; it was only after Christmas that I understood that my teeth were a problem. It was a shock to my system when I realised I had damaged my teeth in the fall and was constantly on painkillers. I thought the problem would go away, but it didn't improve. My GP told me to go to the dentist, but quite a joke that turned out to be. When the private dentist was told my condition, and that I could have a seizure or stroke, they would not take me on. Because of the insurance problems they would not even give me a painkiller.

I was constantly coming across problems with the medical profession due to the fact that I was the one in a million. Nobody had the answers because before me they had never had the questions. I was like a walking guinea pig or a walking time bomb. I found that the only one who could come up with possible answers was the one who understood the questions – me!

I spent eighteen months making many visits to the hospital audio department because I was having trouble with my hearing and my balance. Due to my skull problem, loss of balance could be fatal. The audio department checked and adjusted my hearing aids, but, as I kept telling them, the aids were not faulty; it was something else. I think they thought I was being awkward – after all, I looked so normal. Then I finally got to see a very old consultant. 'Not much hope!' I thought when I met him, but he listened to what I said then put me through some physical tests, which I carried out correctly. Then he told me he had come across this once before many years ago, and he told me what he considered the problem was. It was exactly what I had been saying all along, but nobody had believed me. When I damaged my head the part of the brain connected to my ear had been damaged. Sounds could still enter my ear and be transmitted to my brain, but, because the connection was damaged, the brain could not always process the information properly. When there was a lot of noise it became a confused jumble, I lost my balance and became agitated.

At last I had found someone who understood me – that was the good news. The bad news was there was no solution or cure that the consultant knew of.

Because my GP had become totally confused by visits and questions about something he did not have a clue about he referred me to a clinical physiologist. I turned up at the clinic and told the receptionist my name and whom I had come to see, and I instantly noticed her surprised expression.

She made a call and a few minutes later a lady turned up and, looking surprised, asked, "You are Mr Hughes?"

"Yes," I said.

She looked strangely at me and asked me to wait in a room she took me to. "Mr Turner will be with you in a moment. Please take a seat."

She left me there for a long time, and I got to the stage where I assumed no one was coming and I might as well go home. Then a man came in holding the usual folder. He looked at me very strangely then sat down. From his body language, I could tell he had a problem.

He asked, "You are Mr Hughes?"

"Yes," I said, and I continued telling him a few details, which he scribbled down.

Then he told me why it had taken him so long. After reading my folder he had been trying to work out how to communicate with me. Apparently my turning up as I did confused everybody because normally a person with a folder of information like mine would be in a wheelchair with two carers and have very limited communication with the world. He did say later in our conversation that there was no help he could give me because I knew more about myself and my problems than he could ever imagine. But he did give me some help: at my request he referred me to the dentist at the clinic.

I can never thank the dentist and his staff enough for the help and support they gave me in my many visits. The problems I had were again because of the brain damage. Going to the dentist was completely new to my brain. It was just as though it was the first time, which made it very difficult to cope with and understand. Luckily the dentist realised the trauma I was suffering, and on each visit he did only a small amount of work. When he extracted a tooth I wasn't letting it go without a fight, and he struggled physically to remove it. I think it hurt him more than me. The dentist told me later that in his time he had witnessed and dealt with several cardiac arrests, so I was in good hands. I hoped he was joking, but I wasn't sure.

I spent Christmas on my own because I had reached a stage where I could never predict just how I would react and it was important that I did not ruin anyone else's Christmas by having what I called a wobble. I seemed to have developed several wobbles, and had graded them from 1 to 5 (1 was the lowest level; 5 meant I should be calling for an ambulance). Usually when I woke up in the morning it would take a few minutes to stabilise while I sat up, then another few minutes when I stood up, before I could move off and start the day. During the day I would suffer several wobbles, which could be triggered by any event which happened outside my body.

Because of the problems my abnormal reactions cause others I have produced an accident card. On the front it discloses the state of my skull and gives a list of family contact phone numbers; on the back it discloses the reaction they may see. I realised the need for this information to be available after I visited the local ambulance station to thank them for their help on the day of my accident. We discussed the worry I had that if I had a problem when out and about the normal reaction would probably be that I was drunk or on drugs, and I was told it would be helpful if I carried a card, especially with regard to my skull being open and the brain not covered. The card is to help to insure that if I get into trouble I will be treated correctly and the A & E department will be informed of my condition as soon as I arrive.

I have also been able to find out why doctors and consultants seemed so distant and unsure whenever I visited them. It seemed as though they could never understand what I was talking about and they never have a solution to any of my difficulties. It wasn't totally because they didn't know the answers; it was also because of what had happened to others with similar head injuries. In the USA a man with a similar injury to mine was treated in hospital then woke up and behaved in much the same way as I did, was discharged and looked after himself just as I was doing. People reacted to him in much the same way as they were reacting to me. Then about two months later he dropped dead. The medical explanation is that when the brain is damaged the parts which operate the heart and keep you alive may not recover so successfully as other parts; so you may look as if you have recovered and behave quite normally, but the heart could fail at any time without any warning. When I found this out it made me more aware of my own limited ability to diagnose myself. I had been so agitated at times because my condition was not improving, but I realised that my progress was limited by the damage done to my brain and its ability to recover. I needed to accept that the constant pressure I was applying to myself to return to my former level of health was itself impeding that recovery.

It is very hard for me to accept this. Before my accident I was able to do and achieve so much more than most, and now I have to stand back and watch others carry out jobs which I used to find so easy. It is very difficult for me to accept that the way I can live my life is probably the best it can ever be.

CHAPTER THREE

BACK TO WORK, FEBRUARY 2006

I returned to a full-time job six months after my accident, and I was soon installing equipment to help me with the high-up heavy work because of my balance problems.

On the Headway charity's website they refer to someone they call 'amazing' because five years after his head injury he was able to do a job for a couple of hours a day in a wheelchair.

At Christmas I had cooked an amazing dinner for myself, with all the trimmings, fit for a king, but when I had sat down and had my fill I became very emotionally upset. I reached the lowest ebb of life. I could not taste or even smell my dinner and could not understand why.

I thought I was expecting too soon for things to be back to normal, but when I visited the consultant at Derriford he told me the taste and smell would have returned quite quickly if it was going to, but as it had not returned it probably never would. I was shocked when he told me there was nothing they could do to repair it.

Then came another shock. If I sneeze or cough my brain balloons out through the hole in my skull; I was constantly having weird sensations if a piece of material brushed the side of my head, if I stood with my right side against the wind, if I moved my jaw, if I laughed, etc., etc. I had hoped the hole would just heal up – not so! The consultant at Derriford informed me that he still had my piece of skull which he could put back, or he could fit a metal plate. 'Great!' I thought – but not so! He explained that because of the time factor the skin on my head had stuck itself to my brain, which meant they would have to scrape it off. Now came the bad news: the scraping could cause me to have a seizure or a stroke, which could mean I would be paralysed and in a wheelchair for the rest of my life. He said that in his opinion there was a fifty per cent chance of that happening. The choice was mine to have the operation, he said – but no, there was not much choice. So I have a hole in my skull and have to be very careful. A simple tap could be fatal.

Normally your brain can move around in your skull and react and support balance, etc., but that doesn't happen in my case. I have a problem when I go round bends, etc. My brain is stuck in one position inside my skull and it doesn't move or react in the normal way. If the sun is hot and my brain receives the heat with no protection, it gives me a weird and desperate feeling.

The normal procedure is that when a piece of skull is removed the piece is put back and stapled soon after the surgery is completed. This is what happened in my case, but when they discovered I had MRSA the piece was removed again; and because I had so many problems and was not expected to live it was never put back. I now have to live as I am. To protect the right side of my head I wear a hard hat most of the time. I also find that in bed I have to sleep on my left side. If the right side of my head (and consequently my brain) rests on the pillow, I feel uncomfortable and have to turn over. If I stand without a hat so that the right side of my head is facing towards the wind I get a weird and uncomfortable sensation which causes me to lose my balance and fall over. This can even be caused by the wind from a passing bus or lorry, so I have to ensure I always walk with the road on my left side.

CHAPTER FOUR

MEMORY LOSS

On 7 September I was in an ambulance being transferred back to Torbay. I woke up strapped to a trolley and tried to take in everything around me. I was not able for some reason to move my head, so I used my eyes to look around. To my left the window was frosted, but there was a space I could see through at the top and I noticed we were passing a gantry sign saying, 'Welcome to Plymouth'. My engineering brain registered the equipment as I scanned the interior of the ambulance. Then I noticed a paramedic sitting on the trolley on the opposite side and I studied him for a while, but I didn't remember him from anywhere. It must have been a few minutes before he realised I was looking at him.

He never said a word so I said, "What am I doing here?"

He replied, "You bumped your head, so we are taking you back to Torbay."

I just said, "Oh," and must have gone back to sleep.

I must have woke and slept during the journey as I remember thinking that the only reason I would be in Plymouth was to see Phillip, who was at university. I had arranged to pick him up the next week to take him to Stansted, but of course it was not the second week of August; it was a month later. I had missed a month from my life and had no recollection about that at that moment. I worked out that the ambulance was taking me back home and remembered I was out of milk and would have to pop down to the shop when they dropped me off.

I was awake when we stopped, and I saw when the door was opened that we were at Torbay Hospital, but that didn't bother me. I put that down to Health & Safety and worked out that they had brought me to the hospital to be checked over by the doctor. I was expecting them to then take me home, and I was even more sure of that when they unloaded me and I was put in a side room and not a ward. To me that meant I would not be staying. I did not know this isolation was because of the MRSA. The paramedics were handing over a folder which was about twelve inches thick to the sister, and I knew it could not be related to me because I had only banged my head a few hours before. I assumed it was just some inter-hospital paperwork. I was sure I would just have to wait for the doctor to come round and give me the all-clear and I could go home.

I had no sense of time. When Sheila turned up I let her know I was just waiting for the doctor, then she could give me a lift home; it seemed strange to me when her face looked so surprised and she didn't know what to say.

I have never had any memory about the time I spent at Derriford or the trauma suffered by family and friends or any memory of my fall. I can remember 3 August, the day before my accident, but nothing from about 4 August till 7 September. It's almost as if that time never existed.

It was to be many months before I realised just how long I had been in hospital, and even today I have not come to terms with how critical my injury was and still is. I was told by the consultant that it is normal after an accident for the brain to blank out any of the bad happenings; some can come back or nothing at all.

I look and seem quite normal, yet I can suddenly become distressed and agitated and suffer with emotional storms. This reaction can frighten persons as they think I am having a fit or a heart attack.

CHAPTER FIVE

REACTIONS

During my time at Newton Abbot Hospital my main concern was to get home. It was so very difficult for me. I was treated by medical staff, family and friends as if I had a problem, but I could never see that. To me I had just banged my head and I felt, or seemed to myself, all right. I could not understand all the goings-on around me. As I've said before, the conclusion I came to was that I was being punished and kept in hospital for reasons I could not comprehend. I was thinking that I had to comply with all the requirements to prove what I already knew myself, but what no one else could see. Looking back, I can see that they carried out the standard procedure for a patient with a head injury, but there is no procedure for a patient who is different. In this respect, being a one in a million was counterproductive, to my way of thinking.

What I needed was to sit down with a consultant and for him to explain in explicit detail exactly what damage I had sustained; to describe what action had been taken to stabilise the damage, with details and reactions to all the operations carried out on me; and to set out how I could help to repair myself. Having been a senior design engineer in industry, I was conversant with electrical, mechanical and chemical engineering and was probably more knowledgeable in most fields than most consultants in their fields. I have been very surprised by the lack of knowledge of the workings of the brain, but at least, thanks to my own research, I now have a better understanding of what happened to me.

I have mentioned that I always carry a card, but it is a card I had to design as there was not such a card obtainable from the medical profession. After monitoring my own blood pressure and producing a complex chart to show my GP, he was able to see how to adjust my medication. I see that GPs are now following my method and allowing patients to monitor their own blood pressure. It is just simple common sense that a patient's blood pressure is totally different at home from what it is after an hour and a half in a GP's or hospital waiting room.

It sometimes seems as though the medical profession relies too much on first impressions. That is their downfall. If you look OK, you are OK. Just like the advert, what's on the outside of the tin is what's on the inside. That's OK if you are blind and have a white stick, or if your legs don't work and you are in a wheelchair – many of these kinds of problems have an advert. Perhaps I should have a sign hanging round my neck: 'Head case – approach with extreme caution'.

During the past six years, the reactions of other people have been a constant problem. This is mainly because I appear to be well. No one can realise just how bad I may be feeling at that moment; my reactions may seem frightening and threatening, whereas at that moment I just need help and support. That is why I carry a card explaining my condition – hopefully it will be helpful to persons if I become agitated.

CHAPTER SIX

LIFE SINCE MY ACCIDENT

The six years since my accident passed quickly. I still have no recollection of what happened to me while I was in Derriford Hospital, and that has never been explained totally. I know my accident could have been fatal; I know the operations probably saved my life. So it seems ironic that I could have died from the MRSA infection that the hospital gave me.

When I attended Torbay Hospital for more tests, one was at the Nuclear Medicine Department, where they pumped radioactive fluid into me while I pedalled to increase the pressure so the fluid travelled faster. However, again they assumed I was just another patient so they never told me not to pedal too hard. The rev counter went off the scale and they had to react quickly to stop the machine overloading. The nurse told me later that normally patients need help to turn the pedals round.

When I attended the fracture department regarding my finger I was X-rayed and the consultant explained that he would need to cut the finger off then fix it back with a screw system. This seemed fine, but then he told me the finger would be permanently fixed at right angles. When I got home and sat down and thought about what he had said I could not believe that was the best he could do. My finger would stick out all the time, and that would make putting clothes on, etc. difficult. So I wrote a letter declining his operation. Since then I have worked on my finger myself and have improved it. It is not as good as new, but it is a damn sight better than the consultant suggested.

In 2006 I was convinced that it would take only a few weeks for me to get back to normal. My head was constantly at war with the medical profession. I found it so difficult that day after day would go by and nothing seemed to be happening to improve my problems. This to me was made worse by the attitude of doctors and consultants. None of the ones I visited or was referred to seemed to understand the problems I suffered.

Also in 2006 several deaths occurred at work. Valued colleagues I had worked with for many years lost their lives to cancer or heart failure. Even more upsetting was the loss of a lovely year-six girl to meningitis. During a Friday-afternoon physics lesson she complained of a headache and took a painkiller, and we found out on Monday that she had been taken into hospital and had died on Sunday afternoon. I felt guilty that I had survived my trauma.

By February 2007 two more persons were diagnosed with stomach cancers: one died in 2010 and one is still alive.

Another traumatic year followed in 2011. I lost five more relations of different ages. In August, just a few days before his birthday, my brother Peter left us for no apparent reason – an event that is still very upsetting.

In 2007, despite all the tests I underwent, time went by with no improvement, and in 2008 I bitterly retired from work. I was not able to retire gracefully and sit down like most. Because of my problems I am not able to live in a normal way. I constantly have emotional storms, 'lock-outs' and flashbacks, which make it hard to look after myself properly.

Back in 2005 when I first left hospital I was in a deep trauma because I thought I would be considered unable to look after myself and would end up in a nursing home. That has been a constant worry for me. There have been many times when I should have asked for help, but suffered because I did not want to put on people and spoil their lives or end up in a home.

Because I look and appear so normal when out and about, people sometimes even approach me for help and advice, but who can help me? Who would actually know *how* to help me? In the supermarket persons ask me questions because they think I am the manager, but I may be having a serious wobble and need medical help. But I have to cope. If I were to show what I was feeling inside, I know people would think I was drunk or on drugs and I would be arrested and thrown in a cell for many days. When I get home I sometimes have to sit down and stabilise. This can take between two and five hours, or even a couple of days. I probably would be grateful if I had someone to be with me to help – make a cup of tea, show some understanding, give sensible advice . . . But it is extremely difficult to ask for help because most of the time the help I need is impossible to describe in a way that persons can understand or even respond to. And I can understand that, so I never bother. I often think just how nice it would be to have a person who was more like the person I am without the bang on the head – someone who would understand and react in the way I would react. Persons have often said that I am too complicated for them to understand or relate to. I know that it is extremely difficult for a person to understand something they have never experienced themselves; even those who are classed as experts in their field can only make a guess at a solution.

In April 2012 I visited Brixham Archery Club to see if I could take up archery again. Twenty-five years before I had been the master bowman at an archery club in Oxfordshire and had been the chief coach, and I was hoping I would remember how I was in those days. I have tried using basic equipment and have received extraordinary help, understanding and support. Picking up the bow after twenty-five years seemed totally natural – just as if it was yesterday when I last did it – and my first three arrows were gold. I am now feeling confident enough to take my own equipment, to try and see if I am able to use more powerful equipment. I am expecting to have some problems caused by the 'archery' part of my body being dormant for so long and the muscles being weaker than they were.

I am not sure just how my brain will react to the extra loading. The sport could put additional physical pressure on parts of my brain. This is again an unknown as no one has ever reached this stage before. The standard I had reached in my life before my accident was considerably higher than the norm. I believe that had I just been a normal person I would have either died or ended up as a vegetable in the way most do, but whether I can return to the same level as before is another matter. The physical side is not such a problem as the mental side.

Many times I have felt I will have to go along with the medical profession's prognosis and accept that this is as good as it gets, but I have not yet been able to totally accept that fact. I keep pushing myself. I mean, how exactly do I know when I have reached the limit? Do I just collapse and expire? Again, no one seems to know. I sometimes feel quite despondent when I ask a doctor if it would be OK to do something, and the answer is "Don't know." I can only find out for myself.

In other words: if I try and succeed, it is OK; if I try and collapse and expire, I shouldn't have tried it; if I have a problem and survive, I shouldn't do it again.

Many times in the early night hours I have woken up in a fierce panic, coughing and choking because my throat and airways have become blocked by the mucus leaking from my nose. I spend frightening minutes on my knees trying to clear the blockage and breathe. I take a nose spray when I go to bed and arrange my sleeping position so I am as upright as possible, but it still happens. It feels as though my head will explode. After these attacks I usually can't sleep again, and this gives me what I call a bad day. It takes a while to stabilise and become 'normal' again. By 'normal' I mean able to carry out my usual daily routine, which is difficult owing to the brain being strangled and traumatised while I fought to stay alive. At these times I have no help; no one understands that I need help. But even if I had someone with me, would they understand and be able to help? I have had to come to terms with the thought that if I do expire while at home, it will take probably a few days or weeks before I am discovered. At the same time I realise that fact will not be of concern to myself – only to the persons left behind. After all, they will have to deal with the situation without my being able to assist in any way. When it happens I will probably have no warning. Maybe I will just go to sleep and not wake up again. This is a comforting thought. It takes away the fear of dying.

My father always said, "When you are born the clock inside you starts ticking, and one completely unexpected moment the spring will wind down and the clock will just stop, so don't waste your life watching the clock and waiting; you will, if you are lucky, never know."

CHAPTER SEVEN

THE BEGINNING

I was born in October 1945 at a private nursing home in Leicestershire. My birth sign is Scorpio, which is the most powerful sign, and that fact might have a bearing on the type of person I am. Nothing is known regarding why exactly I was born in a private nursing home; my five brothers were all born at home and all apart from John were christened at Enderby Church in Leicestershire.

I was christened at the church of St Mary de Castro in Leicester. This is strange because it was totally out of context with my parents' lifestyle.

I was also larger at birth than any of my brothers. I weighed in at 10.5 pounds, which caused comments from the midwife; also the vicar, surprised at the weight, nearly dropped me in the font.

The first real change in my life took place when I was just three years old: my brother Terry, who was five, was killed in a road accident on his way home from school.

Stewart was born in December of the same year, followed by the twins two years later. We moved to a small house in Enderby, then to a brand-new larger house.

When I was eight we moved to Southall, Middlesex; when I was fourteen we moved to Bristol; when I was fifteen we moved to Wembley, then to Eastcote. That was our last family house.

My brothers, apart from John, were all married before I was. My first house was in High Wycombe, Buckinghamshire. I undertook many improvements to this house. I designed and installed micro-bore central heating. Because this system was so new in Britain I had to use my lathe to make some of the parts needed; the electrical wiring was completed to comply with the latest IEE regulations.

In the front room I built a new fireplace with extensions to both sides. I decided to use York stone. Most of the rooms were redecorated. The garden was landscaped, new fences were put up and new pathways and a new shed were built. The shed was fitted with equipment for carpentry and metalworking. The smallest bedroom was fitted with a drawing board to enable me to produce drawings for others.

When our first child, Gregory, was born we moved to Rayners Lane, not far from where I worked, to reduce my travelling distance every day.

From there we moved to the village of King's Sutton near Banbury, and in 1988 we moved on to Torquay (my present house).

The second house (at Rayners Lane) was upgraded in many ways. Again the smallest bedroom was set up as a drawing office, and in the front room an engraving machine was set up in the corner. The orchard at the bottom of the garden was levelled off and a forty-foot garage was built and divided in two. One part was a garage with a pit; the other part was a workshop for wood, metal and electrical control-panel assembly. I also installed a complex alarm system to my own design to ensure the firearms safe boxes were protected in accordance with police requirements. During my time at Rayners Lane I was connected to the Metropolitan Police, teaching the use of firearms. I enjoyed archery, league badminton and squash. Related to my work I also worked three nights a week at a technical college, lecturing on industrial and commercial refrigeration to City and Guilds level.

CHAPTER EIGHT

YEARS FLASHING BY

At the age of eleven, using my own resources I became a proficient bike rider and engineer, able to repair and maintain the bicycle that was bought for me by my Uncle Ron, my father's brother. Using this bike I was able to cycle from Southall (West London) to Southend and to Enderby to revisit the area and see the friends I grew up with until we moved to Southall when I was nine. After a fire at the large flat where we lived in Southall, my father's company rehoused us in a similar flat in Kenton, Harrow. I used my bicycle to travel back to Southall to attend my school, (Featherstone County) and the Church Lads' Brigade (CLB); I remained at the school but left the CLB because of the travelling. As there was no CLB in the Kenton area I considered joining the local Scouts, but after a few visits I found that their standard of discipline was not as good as I had become used to at the CLB, so I did not join.

I was already used to riding long distances, and during the summer school holiday I cycled from Kenton to Portsmouth, where I stayed the night in a youth hostel. Next day I went by ferry to the Isle of Wight, and spent the day cycling all over the island. At night I stayed at the Cowes youth hostel. The next day I took the ferry to Lymington and rode through the New Forest, then along the coast to my next youth hostel in an old mill at Bridport, Dorset. From there I cycled on to Lyme Regis, then inland to the A4 at Marlborough, turned east and cycled back to London, arriving back home in the early hours. My mother got up and cooked me a breakfast. I had been away for some ten days.

My family never really knew where I had been during the time I was not at home. I had sorted out the route myself, written to and booked the youth hostels, sending postal orders from money made from jobs, sorted out my clothing, bought and fitted panniers to the rear of the bicycle, packed cleaning materials and spares for the bike and just cycled off and back. In Southampton a bracket on one of the panniers had broken. I found a cycle shop, and the kind owner welded and repaired the bracket at no cost and wished me luck on my travels.

Reading cycling magazines, I was captivated by stories relating to the Tour de France – so much so, that at the age of twelve I traded in my Hercules bicycle with the Sturmey-Archer gears and dynamo hub, and used the money I had saved from all my jobs to buy a Claud Butler racing bicycle. I joined a cycling club and cycled many miles with other club members. Despite being the youngest by some ten years I was able not only to keep up but to outperform them all. At the same time I learnt that physical ability was not the same as mental ability; and despite some being very good at pointing that out to me, there were some who were very helpful and enjoyed teaching me. Thank you!

There were some design deficiencies with the bicycle I was using, so I produced sketches of the improvements I wanted. I then took my frame and sketches to Fred Perry, a former racing cyclist who was now retired and running his own cycle shop near Wembley. After I had discussed my sketches with him he agreed to help. He was able to send my frame to Holdsworthy, a company that made cycles, and their design department carried out the work and produced the frame I required. Later Fred Perry told me that the boss of Holdsworthy told him that my frame was the most complex design they had ever seen, and he was astonished when Fred told him I was only thirteen years old. The main reason my design was different to the normal was because of its inner strength. With the normal design the frame would bend under stress – not break, but whip, as it was called. Some riders liked that, but I realised that energy and power were being lost between the rider and the road. It was a waste. In my design all the lugs which keep the tubing together were strengthened, as were the wheel-mountings, the frame ends and the bottom-bracket housing. The front forks were normally made from oval tubing, but on my frame I changed this to round tubing. This increased the frame's rigidity and strength. I selected all the frame components using my own engineering knowledge and understanding. Most of the components were made in Italy, a country of many years of cycling achievements. The wheel hubs were Campagnolo quick-release; the headstock was Campagnolo fitted with English bearings. At that time the normal seat was English – Brooks leather – but I thought that was old-fashioned and heavy, so I obtained a nylon lightweight seat from Italy. The design was very similar to the ones now in use on the 2012 Tour de France. The rear-wheel gear sprockets were English; the gear changers, rear and front, were Campagnolo; the gear levers fitted into the ends of the handlebars so that you could change gear without removing your hands from the bars. This was essential if you were head down, sprinting. The cranks, also from Italy, were longer than normal to give more leverage. They were fitted with special bolt locking to prevent them coming loose.

Most of the items were sourced and imported by Fred Perry. This was because a lot of the items were not normally available in this country. Luckily I was able to gleam information from studying the bikes used on the Tour de France, and I agreed with Fred that when he obtained the parts he could display them in his shop for a couple of weeks before I used them. When I obtained the Mafac Tiger brakes they caused quite a stir. Many of the other bike riders had heard about them, but they had never actually seen them before. When I completed the bike I agreed to display it in Fred's shop on a Saturday if I was working elsewhere. In this way I could repay him not just for his help and support but for allowing me to pay my bill weekly. Otherwise it would have taken a very long time to complete my project. Fred, thank you!

One of the many jobs I undertook was working in the bakeries where my father was the chief engineer. I did this from the age of eleven. When the normal bakery employees took their holidays, my father would get me work as a replacement. I worked in each department as required and learnt most aspects of the trade. By the time we moved to Bristol I was quite a proficient worker and carried on doing the same at the Bristol bakery. Sometimes I would work a twelve-hour day shift and carry on with a twelve-hour night shift. I hardly ever saw daylight! Pay was cash in hand and about £1 an hour, so I was able to give my mother some and save for the items I needed. Nowadays, all this working would not be allowed because of my age, and Health & Safety.

Moving to Bristol was quite a change for me. When Mr Downs, the head teacher at Featherstone, was told I was moving he interviewed me and told me that it would be better if I could stay at Featherstone to complete my education as he did not know of any suitable schools in the Bristol area. But because of the cost and non-availability of any family connections it was not possible for me to stay on – a decision that would be against me at a later time.

A few weeks later, when we arrived in Bristol, I had to visit the Bristol education offices. When I entered the office of the person I had to see I could tell from his body language that I was not being welcomed with open arms. The reason was soon apparent. He drummed his fingers on the letter in front of him and told me it was a letter from Mr Downs stating my requirements for my education. It was then pointed out that the only school that would meet Mr Downs' criteria was in the city of Bath, which was outside the Bristol area. For me to attend that school would mean a lot of, in his opinion, unnecessary paperwork and my parents would have to fund the transport. I knew I could cope with all the travelling, but there was no way my parents could provide the money for transport and clothing. I understood about the cost of bringing up five boys, and it was impossible for me to fund myself, so I agreed to attend a school fairly local to where we lived in Bedminster: Ashton Park. I rode past the school at the weekend and it looked like a nice location. But – oh, boy! – on Monday when I turned up and joined the other children entering the premises the initial shock for me was that there were girls. Having just spent five years at a boys-only school, girls were totally alien to me. Good grief! Girls didn't do woodwork, engineering or drawing; they didn't play football, cricket, rugby or basketball; they didn't ride bikes. And if you compare netball with basketball— Well, I ask you! There's simply no comparison. Later, when some of us boys played hockey against a girls' team the boys all ended up covered in bruises from being hit with the hockey sticks wielded by the girls. They took advantage of our kind and sporting nature.

The second shock was the standard of teachers, and the lack of facilities and equipment. At Featherstone the teachers had served time in proper jobs before becoming teachers. Morgan, the engineering teacher, had been an aircraft engineer, so not only did we have a fully equipped workshop, but he taught us about proper engineering, even including case-hardening of materials, and I had become a proficient machine operator. I had spent a considerable time making components for Mr Morgan's pet project: the making of his own car using the bodywork from a Jowett Javelin and an old Spitfire engine. We had a fully equipped drawing office with parallel motion set up on every desk. One teacher was a former chief draughtsman; the woodwork teacher was a former cabinetmaker for Parker Knoll; the art teacher had had some of his paintings hung in national galleries. We also had a full-size pottery kiln and a ceramics department. Mr Evans, the geography teacher, had spent time walking the world. He could teach from his own knowledge and experience and not just from a textbook. By the time I was in the second year the new school building had been completed and the new Featherstone was the first school in Middlesex to have a colour television set. The new gym had a sprung wooden floor; the cricket pitch had an all-weather wicket; the dining room had a modern kitchen; the building had proper indoor toilets. The English teacher, Miss Wilks, looked at least 100 years old, but she commanded total respect. She would spend time talking with each pupil about his essay, pointing out the good points and explaining the bad points. She taught us proper English and the correct way to use it. The sports teacher had years of experience working for professional clubs, etc., etc.

So when I observed the classroom facilities and met the teachers at Ashton Park I felt dismayed, but I realised I would have to make the best of it and make it work for me. In some ways it was the start of a different life. I found that instead of learning from teachers I was teaching the teachers, and because of that I became more knowledgeable about others and myself – and I quickly learnt that nobody likes a smart alec.

The English teacher at Ashton Park spent a whole lesson giving out the book to read for the exam. This was *Pride and Prejudice*. We were then told to read a page every week. At the next lesson he started to explain what the author's thoughts were. I put my hand up to contradict what he had said and referred to many pages in the book to justify my thoughts. He tried to disclaim my theories by asking just how many pages I had read, so I informed him that I had read the entire book. He looked shocked and asked just how long that took me. I told him two hours. He quickly dismissed the subject and moved on to another topic. I don't think he ever spoke or acknowledged me ever again, which was disappointing because I wasn't trying to undermine him; I wanted him to be helpful and teach me. After all, that is what he was paid to do!

While I lived in Bristol, on Sunday mornings I would deliver newspapers for a local shop. At that time the Sunday paper had just started to include magazines, etc., which made the paper bag too heavy for the other boys to carry, so I took on the deliveries. One day, after completing the deliveries and returning the bag to the shop, the shopkeeper informed me that there was someone who wanted to see me. My immediate thought was that perhaps I had delivered the wrong papers or damaged one when posting it, but the man waiting in the back room introduced himself as Eddy Cuttle and he seemed pleased to see me. He was the manager of an amateur football club called Exeter City, and the man who scouted for him had given him my name as a promising player. The reason for the secret meeting in the back room was explained to me: because I was still a schoolboy he wasn't officially allowed to approach me. He explained that if I was interested in playing at a higher level than my present school level, I would have to appear to approach him; so the following Saturday morning I went to see the team playing and asked Eddy if I could play.

I started to play there regularly and was able to adapt quite quickly to playing with men of twice my age. I experienced a lot of animosity from other players – especially members of teams we played. Eddy had warned me that most men would not be pleased that a young kid was probably a better player than they were. In one match, despite playing in defence at right back, I was able to set up the centre forward to score two goals. In another match I got so fed up with the forwards not scoring that I moved forward and scored three goals to show them how to do it. My exploits were not appreciated by all the players, but I enjoyed playing at this level and stayed with the club until my family moved to Wembley.

The year I spent at Ashton Park was my last school year, so at the end of July I started to look for a job. I had set my heart on being a draughtsman, but before I could attend any interviews my father announced that we were moving again. He had got a job with better prospects than his present job. My father was a very good bakery engineer and was held in high esteem by Baker Perkins, which supplied most of the bakeries in the UK with equipment. Because of his capabilities and experience he was often referred to companies who were looking for an experienced engineer; as such he never had to apply for a job. He explained to me that he had been offered a job with better pay and conditions and he said it would be better for my youngest brother, John, who had developed asthma. Where we lived in Bristol was near the river and that made the area damp and not good for John, but we could have quite easily moved away from the river basin if he had wanted to stay in Bristol.

Our new location was Wembley, which meant I could easily cycle to Southall to meet up with the friends I had left behind when we moved to Bristol. It was good to be able to forget the Bristol intrusion into my life.

I found a job working at Eldwood's, a refrigeration company on the trading estate behind Wembley Stadium, and it was right next to the bakery complex where my father worked. He was given a company car, so I was able to have a lift to and from work. While at Eldwood's I trained as a draughtsman, attended day release at technical college and read refrigeration at City and Guilds level. I gained a first-class pass and was awarded a prize for the highest marks ever recorded.

Eldwood's was then taken over by another company and I experienced the methods used by property developers: despite all their spoken promises it was soon evident that their real interest was the land and not the business. Eldwood's was closed down and the equipment was sold off. That was hardest for the persons who had been there for many years and were too old to get other jobs. Some of the workers had been there when Mr Eldwood came over from America, and they had helped him set up the business; some had been there during the Second World War, and had been working at their machines making components for aeroplanes for the war effort as the bombs were dropping around them. The War Ministry had delivered sheets of corrugated metal to put over their workplaces, to protect them. That's what the man from the ministry said! They pointed out to me that if a bomb had landed 100 feet away they were goners, so the corrugated metal was just useless propaganda. Luckily, because of my grades at college and my reputation, I was headhunted by another refrigeration company; so I walked out of the door at Eldwood's and in a door at Prestcold. This was a definite move in the right direction as it was a larger company with better prospects, and it was operating in a much wider market.

During this time I reached twenty-one and was given a quite lavish party by my parents to celebrate my birthday and my engagement to Jennifer. I was busy saving to get married and have a house and 2.4 children – that was the normal life to aim for, so everyone told me – so I had several other jobs as well as my day job.

One of these jobs was repairing cars. I could take the engine, or gearbox, or back axle out of most cars – repair, rebuild, replace. I was also proficient at panel-beating and respraying. Most of the tools I used were of my own design and manufacture. In those days you could only charge half a crown an hour, which meant it took eight hours to make a pound. I could buy a gallon of Duckhams 20–50 engine oil for twelve and six and charge fifteen shillings to make a profit.

When I bought my first house I had £1,500 in the building society; the buying price of the house was £4,500; the salary from my day job was £1,600 a year. At the time petrol was cheaper than four gallons for £1 and your car was filled for you and your windscreen cleaned. At cheap pubs, chicken, chips and a glass of wine cost £1; fish and chips cost two and six (half a crown). You think: eight meals for a pound! That's better value than nowadays. My first day job had a salary of £5.50 a week, which was good compared with the salaries of my friends from school. At that time a married man with children would be lucky to earn £10 to £12 a week; a rise was good if it was twenty-five pence an hour.

When I left school my priorities were job, money, transport. I decided to get a scooter or motorbike, then save for a car. A car was the ultimate because with a car you could dress smart and take people out, instead of having to wear waterproofs and winter clothes. Also on a motorbike or scooter, because of the mod-and-rocker problems, you were likely to be stopped and searched every couple of miles by the police. You could be stopped many times by the same policeman. If I was riding along and saw a policeman, I stopped and laid out my documents on the seat for when he got to me. Some policemen would be pleased and smile; some would growl, thinking I was being clever.

On a Friday night the norm after working all week was to watch *Ready Steady Go!* on the television. Then we would all meet at Burtons in Uxbridge. The tailor's had a dance hall over the shop. Usually the boys would gather round the outside of the dance floor, talking about things that were important to them like clothes, work, cars, bikes, pop stars, etc. The girls would be dancing round their handbags, hoping a boy would ask for a dance. The boys would watch, hoping another would be the first to take the plunge. When the musicians went off for a smoke records would be played. If you spotted a girl you fancied, you waited until they put on the Animals' record 'The House of the Rising Sun' – not because of the music or words, but because that was the longest record in the world. Mind you, it could go against you if the girl you fancied turned out to be the opposite to your hopes and expectations. Then the record would seem to go on for ever.

The girls were mad on hairspray to keep their hair in shape; so if you were dancing and your heads met, her hair felt like concrete. And all the girls had the same smell.

At the end of the evening it was a mad ride back to be first in the queue at the fish-and-chip shop in Adelaide Road, Southall. My favourite was rock salmon and chips, bread and butter, and a cup of tea. We would stay there till the shop closed.

I always worked during the day on Saturday, but in the evenings we might drive to Bognor Regis and back or go to stock-car racing at Wimbledon.

Sunday was another workday for me, but I would socialise in the evening.

My friends moved up to cars before me, but that was because they all bought old bangers. I knew they were bangers because I was the one who repaired them. I didn't want to buy an old banger, so I saved for longer and bought a 1959 Riley to replace my scooter.

I had been courting Jennifer, a sister of a boy I had been to school with but was not a close friend of. Alan was always just Jennifer's brother. During the time I became close to Jennifer and her family there were lots of reasons why I should not have considered marriage, but at that age I thought any problems would sort themselves out and disappear when we were married. If the problems were so obvious, then maybe I thought Jennifer would decline; as she didn't, things must be OK. Unfortunately some time after the wedding Jennifer told me she had never wanted to get married, and even on the day she had had second thoughts. She went through with it because she was concerned about the way it would upset her mother. In other words, it was more important than how she felt about me. There were three people in my marriage and I was the odd one out.

I should have listened to my dear old granny. After she first met Jennifer, years before we were married, she told me she was a very nice girl but was not right for me. At the time I dismissed the remark – after all, what did my old granny know? – but I have never forgotten her words of wisdom.

Anyway, we discussed divorce quite soon after our marriage, but for some reason we stayed together; and because of this situation I devoted most of my time to work and not play. When I was forty I was told in a conversation with a wise old man that a normal person would have to live 150 years to achieve as much as I had already.

Another change of direction occurred when I was again headhunted. One of the largest British companies was setting up an alliance with a German refrigeration company, and I became their youngest senior design engineer. This was another step in the right direction for me; it was also a very demanding position which would stretch me to my limits and beyond,

I was now carrying out not only design and installation of commercial refrigeration, but also design and installation of refrigeration and air conditioning for industrial food-processing plants. In the latter days at Prestcold I had become involved with industrial plant and had visited the government complex at Aldermaston to design air conditioning for the laboratories so that any air was clean and to prevent contamination. In my new position I was to design large cold-storage units for most of the large companies, such as M&S, Tesco, Sainsbury's, Express Dairies, Quaker Oats, Nestlé's, etc., etc.; food-processing systems for Bernard Matthews, King Harry Foods and Brooke Bond; refrigeration systems for ice-cream manufacturers, medical gas suppliers, blood banks, mortuaries and abattoirs; and special systems for Kellogg International and Monsanto Chemicals (explosion-proof systems). Some of my designs were for export and are probably still in use in faraway places. The export projects were more time-consuming because they usually needed installation and operating manuals, so I had to produce manuals that other persons could actually understand. Diagrams and drawings were essential, and this was in the pre-computer era. Today's designers cannot imagine just how lucky they are to have computer systems. In those days we employed typists who would type from dictation. The lucky ones had electric typewriters; but, even so, to produce a manual would take weeks, and if you made any alterations the typist would have to type the pages again. When finished, the pages with drawings and diagrams would be sent to the printer. Master copies were always kept in my office.

At BOC my boss was an Oxford engineering graduate. His mind was so brilliant that he could write Einstein's theory from memory on the back of a cigarette packet, but he could not boil an egg. He could write down the method and all the calculations to prepare the perfect boiled egg, but didn't know how to put the theory into practice. So whenever he wanted to put into practice an engineering operation he had worked out he would explain it to me and I would write it down clearly and concisely in language the site engineers could understand. He once asked me why it was that I could understand him and convey his meaning to others; yet if he spoke to those same people directly, they could not understand anything he said. To me it was quite simple. I have always said I can speak many languages, but none of them are foreign. I never talk down or up to a person; I adjust my conversation to their level. In this way they never feel overwhelmed or threatened; often they feel important. I know I can appear quite daunting to people who meet me for the first time, so I always try to make sure my manner is pleasant and inviting. But since my accident in 2005 I have not been quite the same and there have been times when I have become frightening and confusing to others. This is because, although physically I look exactly the same as I always did, mentally I am different – completely different.

I did not have the time to complete all our contracts by myself, although at the time it often seemed as though I did. I often spent hours – days! – on the phone, giving instructions, help and advice to installation engineers on sites all over the world. When we obtained a contract I would visit the site, and in my mind I would lay out and install the complete plant. I would then produce sketches and supervise the installation drawings as well as the detailed instructions, making sure that the components were ordered and supplied to the site at the correct time. I also produced operational manuals for the customers' site engineers.

Some of the contracts were covered by Lloyd's or Vulcan insurance, so they had to approve all the drawings. The site installation engineers also had to be approved, and the welders were tested and checked before they could start. If a change was required during the installation, new drawings had to be produced and approved before the change could take place. One of my trainee draughtsmen, John, when he brought me his drawing to approve could not understand how without looking I could tell him the mistakes. That wasn't magic – I would always be the first in the office in the morning, usually two or three hours before others, and

I would go round and look at all the drawings. That is how I knew John's mistakes before he brought his drawing to me. On the day I left BOC, John told me his big aim was to produce a drawing which had no mistakes. I did not ever tell him how I knew his mistakes.

If a contract was for an explosion-proof area, then all the components had to have test certificates to comply with the regulations. For example, a small pressure switch would have to be encased in a Buxton housing, which would make the installation of the item huge. Every complete installation would have to pass all the tests before it could be signed off and handed over.

In my drawing office I employed competent draughtsmen and some trainees, and because of the size of BOC we would have other overseas persons to train as well. The person I remember most fondly was a German girl, Ingrid Carson, whom I employed for her German knowledge and draughtsman skills. Ingrid had come from Hamburg to work in the UK. She was able to carry out translations for a lot of the German design drawings. She had also worked at the German company we were part of. The reason for my fondest memory is simple: she was the only female I have ever met who would have been the perfect wife for me. So why didn't it happen?

Ingrid's parents, who were still living in Hamburg, had put the war and its causes behind them. They would have been quite happy for Ingrid to marry an Englishman, but – and it's a big but – Ingrid had a brother who hated the British. He was two years younger than her, and he was a member of a society in Germany which had rallies and meetings. Its members were mainly young men who hated Hitler because he lost the war, and hated the British and Americans and any others who were related in some way to Germany's defeat. They spent most of their time dreaming of their Germany rising up again and succeeding where Hitler failed. When this brother found out that Ingrid was working in the UK, he was ridiculed by the society and had to convince them that she was working in the UK as a spy and would be useful to their cause; so whenever Ingrid went home she was interrogated by her brother and his friends about the UK. So we knew it would not be possible for her to ever be with an Englishman.

At this time, thanks to the money I had saved from the many different jobs I was doing, we were able to buy our first house, a three-bedroom semi in High Wycombe, Buckinghamshire. This meant travelling early into London to our jobs and arriving back in the late evening. My spare time was used doing drawing work for other companies on a freelance basis, and improving the property to my design. Complete rewiring and the installation of central heating were undertaken. I used a new micro-bore system which was so new that I had to machine new fittings on my lathe as they were not yet available in the UK. In the front room I designed a fireplace with side extensions using York stone ordered from Yorkshire. Other rooms were renovated and decorated, the garden was landscaped, and a workshop was built. The garage was used to build a veranda for my parents' caravan at Selsey. Because my Riley was rusting away I had purchased an old Mini Van, so I rebuilt that and included a new rear subframe, new side windows, new seating, and an improved and upgraded engine system. I then resprayed it – dark-brown metallic.

This was used as our transport for a time; then our next car was a Viva SL90, which was then replaced owing to rusting by a Sunbeam Rapier H120. This was a fast car, having an engine upgraded by Holby. This meant a twin overhead cam engine with twin Weber 40 DCOE carburettors, which in magazine testing had proved to be as efficient as the new fuel-injector system that was starting to be used by some of the more expensive cars of the era. The Rapier was also fitted with overdrive on the top three gears, which meant you did not need to keep putting the clutch down to change gear when travelling fast through country lanes. It was a pillar-less saloon – probably the best car I have owned.

While at High Wycombe Jennifer became pregnant – a fact she was not very pleased about. In fact, she was very annoyed because it meant she would have to give up her job, which was more important to her than having children. After she had got over that thought, she realised that it would please her mother – which was by far the most important factor in Jennifer's life.

Jennifer's mother had a good friend, Mrs Thomas, who had a

daughter the same age as Jennifer. This daughter had also got married, and she had a child, so Mrs Thomas had a granddaughter – a fact we were constantly reminded of. Jennifer's mother was hoping to have a grandchild before she died. She already had a grandson, Mathew, but he was completely cast aside because Jennifer's mother would not tolerate the girl her son had married

I decided to move closer to my workplace so I would not spend so much time travelling to and from work. At work I was already constantly travelling to meetings and for site visits. This idea was accepted by Jennifer and her mother because it would also mean they were closer to each other.

So we sold up and moved to a house in walking distance of my offices. That was good – well, almost. It also meant that Jennifer's parents were often at our home.

Shortly after we moved, our first child, Gregory, was born; a few years later our second child, Heidi, arrived.

The years at Rayners Lane were peppered with many changes to my world. My job was very demanding of my time, knowledge and experience, and I spent many weekdays and weekends on sites around the UK. I also set up various home-based work, engraving signs for control panels, etc., building control panels, carrying out vehicle repairs and fitting spare parts, producing design drawings for companies . . . I was also lecturing (City and Guilds refrigeration) three nights a week at a technical college.

I was a registered firearms certificate holder, and I coached at gun clubs. As a registered shotgun holder I took part in many clay shoots. As a master bowman I coached at an archery club. I played squash and badminton at league level.

I was also a special constable. Many times I would arrive home from work on a Friday evening, have some food, 'kiss and goodbye' the children and be out all night keeping the streets safe. I would return home just as the children got up from their night's sleep. I must admit there were times when I wondered if I had just had my last time at home and I would become another statistic. I would grab a couple of hours' sleep in the afternoon before spending another evening out on patrol. At that time police numbers had fallen owing to low pay and they were considering taking industrial action. This put increased pressure on special constables and their own employment.

I also sometimes spent weekends on installation sites around the country. Some days I would pop over to London Airport and jump on the shuttle service to Scotland, collect a hire car and travel to a site, then fly back to London, arriving home in the late evening. This could happen several times during a single week. At other times I would spend a couple of days at a site for handovers and acceptance, lecturing the customer's engineers with regard to operational service and explaining the repair manuals.

One day the time arrived when I could see no light at the end of the tunnel, so I decided to drop out of the rat race, buy a village general stores and post office and live a proper life.

After many visits and a great deal of searching I found such a property in an Oxford village near Banbury. We purchased it, and the house in Rayners Lane was sold. It was to be a new life – a new beginning.

Everybody was pleased for us – well, not quite everyone. A couple of weeks before the move there was still one person who was not aware of our moving, and that person was Jennifer's mother. Jennifer was frightened about what her mother's reaction would be, and she had not told her despite my encouraging her to do so.

Then I had a call from my mother. She had planned a sort of gathering to wish us well, and unaware that Jennifer's mother had not been told she had rung her to sort out the arrangements. She was flabbergasted by Jennifer's mother's reaction. I then told Jennifer that her mother now knew and how she had found out, so Jennifer went ballistic and called my mother several names. We then had a visit and scene from Jennifer's outraged mother. It was obvious from her reaction that she thought I was to blame for taking her daughter away from her and moving to the other side of the world. She would never see her daughter or her grandchildren again, she said. Actually the distance was about fifty miles.

The scene was a copy of the one when we married and were

leaving the reception: Jennifer's mother held on to her and wouldn't let her go, and some of her relations had to pull them apart so we could leave.

A few days later I was told by Jennifer that her parents were worried that their car would not make the journey to visit us – so could I find a better car? I asked how much they wanted to pay, and I was told they only had £300; so I phoned my brother Paul, who at that time worked for a used-car dealer. He told me I could not get anything useful for that amount of money. A lady I knew at work, Sylvia Peters, had a very nice Viva which was low mileage and not too old. Having done the servicing on it, I knew it was in very good condition. Sylvia had bought it new and was upgrading, so I asked her how much the garage was giving her in part exchange. That was £525, so I asked her if I could buy the car from her at the same price. She said yes because she could get her new car at a lower price without the trade-in.

I asked Jennifer to ask her parents to come over and look at the car. When they saw it they were very pleased – even more so when I told them it was £300. Did they want it? Gosh, yes! So I said if they gave me the money I would give it to Sylvia. That didn't go down well with Jennifer's mother. She was adamant that they would see Sylvia and give her the money. The look on her face said it all: she didn't trust me. After all, I was stealing her daughter, and if I said £300 it was probably only £200. So I said that was OK and I would tell Sylvia that they would contact her. I took the car back to work and told a pleased Sylvia they wanted it. I also told her they thought they were paying £300. I asked her to go along with that and I gave her the £225 difference from my pocket. After the transaction Sylvia told me they were very strange people, and yes, as I had told her, they were very suspicious about the price. They asked a lot of probing questions about me, and Sylvia said she felt like giving them a slap. I had worked many years with Sylvia and many times had helped her out of a difficult situation, so she knew me well.

A few days later I asked Jennifer's parents how the car was. Oh, yes, marvellous! They had been to a car dealer who had an almost identical car, but not in such good condition, and he was asking £585; so it seemed as though they (not I) had negotiated a very good price when they bought it. There was never a thank you in my direction, but they were never ever to know about my deception.

Our new property was 400 years old, and the floors and walls were original. I could see there was an enormous amount of work for me to undertake, and I spent the next ten years upgrading: rebuilding, extending, wiring, plumbing, painting, decorating, etc.

After a few months I realised the difference between the village life and what I had been used to. I felt my brain was going to sleep. I mean, I had moved backwards. I had been working 24/7 in a high-tech environment with top engineers, consultants and architects, but in the village time had stopped. The most important conversation was about the weather, or Mary's bunions. Some of the village persons had been born there and never left – not even for a holiday. Some had never worked. Some could not read or write. There were complete families, living next door to one another or close. Everyone knew all about everyone else.

When I took on the post office, I employed a lady who was a Wyatt. That turned out to be a good move on my part because 'Wyatt' was one of the oldest village names. Sheila Wyatt was a village woman whose husband had died and she had been left to bring up their daughter on her own. My employing her moved me up a few notches on the village 'Who to Like' list. Also Sheila knew everybody and everything and was a very useful person to ensure we did not do the wrong things and upset anybody. We found out that we might have bought the shop but the villagers actually owned it, so we did not make any changes unless we knew they would be accepted. The villagers never liked change unless they believed it was really their idea in the first place.

There were several clubs in the Banbury area, so I was able to carry on with the sporting side of life. I arranged for Jennifer to run the shop and post office several days a week, and I set up a business doing domestic and commercial repairs and installations. Because of my capabilities I built up a growing reputation and soon found I had more and more work – especially with local farms and special pig-breeding units.

Using the extra money I was able to undertake the refurbishment and upgrading of the old property. In ten years the half-acre garden was landscaped and new lawns were laid. The rockery I built was eighty feet long and took hundreds of plants. I grew most of my own plants and also sold them in the shop. On the other side of the garden I built aviaries and breeding units, and I had some 200 birds of different species. The barn was reroofed and had a new level concrete floor, and it was wired. I used it as a workshop for repairs and the manufacture of replacement parts of many types. The main building roof was replaced, and another part of the building had a complete new roof and structure. All the roof space was insulated, covered with felt and re-slated. The building was 100 feet long. Because the roof timbers were original oak, well seasoned and very hard, to put the slate back we needed to use masonry nails. Inside, upstairs, two more bedrooms were built with shower-and-toilet rooms. The original bathroom was rebuilt with new equipment and a separate toilet. Downstairs the main lounge was extended to an L shape. The large inglenook was refurbished with a metal canopy, and we bought an extra-large basket to take the large logs. I spent many a magical evening in front of that fire, feeling the warmth, watching the dancing flames. I remember the wonderful smell when burning applewood. We fitted a new kitchen, a new dining room, and a new front lounge with original inglenook opened up. Many years before, because of the cost of coal, a lot of inglenooks were filled in and replaced with a small grate. To uncover the inglenook took two skip-loads of rubble.

Part of the property extended behind the shop, and I converted this into a guest annex with its own bathroom. Two rooms that had been storerooms I converted into an office and storage area.

A new garage was built at the end of the property. This had to be large enough so I could put the car in and open the car doors on both sides.

The entire property was rewired. Some of the existing wiring was very old and the rubber insulation had perished. The building had been in danger of catching fire for a long time.

The room above the shop was fairly new compared with the rest of the building. This was because there had been a fire many distant years past, but that was before electrical wiring. The fire had occurred when the building had been a bakery. In those days all the villagers had their own pigsties and the room above the shop had been used for storage of hams; so, because of the heat and smoke, the room above the bakery oven was the ham-curing focal point of the village.

During the refurbishment the poor quality of the workmanship of the builders from the distant past became evident. The main walls had no deep foundations and were built of stone held in place with mud and water. There was no proper grouting. It's very similar to drystone walling. To put soil pipes through the wall was easy: just remove the stones by hand. There was a problem, though, when putting in wiring or heating piping; the walls were three to four feet thick so I needed a very long drill. The vibration would loosen the stones, so when I pulled the drill out they would fill the hole. I had to put the drill right through the wall and place a sleeve on the drill so that when I pulled the drill out the sleeve would pull through and remain in the hole. I could then fit the wiring.

Because the kitchen walls were not square there was no way to put up wall cupboards. The flooring was just garden soil, so that was removed and a waterproof membrane was fitted and covered with concrete. To support the wall cupboards I welded up a frame using a goalpost type of structure and bolted it to the floor and wall. The cupboards were very easy to mount on this frame, and I used the void behind for wiring and piping so the finished kitchen looked quite normal and modern.

During our time in the village we had another child, Phillip.

After nearly ten years I reached another thinking time. I could see that the world was changing. I could see that village shops were disappearing. The post-office work was disappearing, as was the income. It was becoming necessary to calculate how best to survive in the future, so I made a decision that we would put the property up for sale. If it sold, we would move; if it didn't sell, we would stay and find more successful sources of income. Another reason for our attempt to move was that Gregory and Heidi had reached a time in their education when a move would not be a problem. They were spending three to four hours travelling by coach to and from school, so we hoped to move to a house closer to their schooling.

The previous year we had spent a week's holiday in Torquay, Devon. When we travelled down on the Saturday the sun was shining – but the travel was horrendous, mainly due to the traffic. The Sunday was overcast. Then it rained from Monday to Friday. Trying to find things for three children to do in the dry was not easy. Then on the Saturday we faced the same journey home traffic-wise. It seemed so silly to spend a year working, book a holiday then find it was more a headache than enjoyment. The solution was quite plain to me: we should live by the coast. If the sun shines, we have a holiday; if it rains, we stay indoors. I investigated the schools in Torquay, and they had a good report. But to be sensible I decided not to buy another property until we had sold and had the money in the bank.

I contacted an estate agent specialising in business premises, and they valued and marketed the village business for us. We had the usual time-wasters, but eventually sold to persons who were moving from Devon; so on the day of the changeover the removal lorry that delivered them also loaded our load for a return trip. Our house contents were stored in Torquay until we found a property. In the meantime we rented a property in Paignton.

Our priority was to settle Gregory and Heidi into school; and they were both accepted by the main grammar schools, which although separated were on the same site. We were then able to find a property within a few minutes' walking distance. This property was a big change: it required hardly any work. All the walls, etc. were straight and level with no horsehair plaster. Even the floors were level. The garden was small, but later I was able to purchase another plot to double the size. Because the property was a great deal smaller than our previous home it seemed a bit cramped, so I had another bedroom built. Now for me it is too big! The location was right. If the sun was shining, we could all pop down and sit on the beach and the kids could swim in the sea. On a Saturday I could stand and watch all the traffic building up as holidaymakers started the long journey home, and I would remember what it had been like.

Since 1988 and the move to Devon there have been many changes to my life. I accepted a position at the grammar school where Heidi was a pupil, and I brought in many changes. At that time schools only had a few BBC computers, but I had been using computers for many years and installed a computer network with miles of cabling over a vast, complex site. When they needed air conditioning, I was able to help with that too. The science labs had very basic old and out-of-date apparatus, so I produced a vast amount of updated apparatus and worksheets. I also built some twenty computer rooms: forty classrooms had projectors, computers and interactive boards fitted. Wireless networks were installed throughout the school. Several server systems and hubs were installed for teaching staff, pupils and the administration department.

Originally the move to Devon was good for the family, but the job situation in Devon is not very good. Gregory went to Cardiff University and obtained a first-class degree. He was able to find a more lucrative job market in the Bristol area. Heidi went to Welbec army sixth-form college, then obtained her degree at the Royal Military College of Science. Part of her degree work involved the design of stab-proof vests, which are in use by security and police forces. She then graduated from Sandhurst. Heidi also spent a year travelling extensively with the royal family and had afternoon tea with the Queen on many occasions. Heidi now has the rank of major. Phillip attended Plymouth University. He now resides in New Zealand, expecting in 2013 to relocate to Canada. Gone are the days when families lived next to each other. The world has changed – so have the habits of people.

Jennifer and I have separated, but we are still good friends. I believe that when you have children you have a responsibility to keep on good terms. After Jennifer's mother died Jennifer became the real person she is. She had spent a good many years of her life being the person her mother wanted: the perfect daughter. Now, with her gone and the children living their own lives, she has been able to do all the things she wanted to do but couldn't without upsetting her mother, or because of the demands of bringing up children. I have been able to dust off the books I started writing so many years ago, and hopefully I can also complete the projects and develop the ideas which were kept dormant by family commitments.

The accident I suffered in 2005 was a big blow to me. I suffered a major setback to my life and lifestyle. Just before 4 August I had been planning to up sticks and move to live in France, but with my life altered so dramatically that doesn't look very practical now. Most importantly, I am still alive, which I am told is a miracle. I take each day as it comes, try to be positive and work as hard as I can to get back on track.

It was a special moment for me when my first book, *Purple Jade,* was published. I hope the story will be well read and show some persons that the apparently easy answers to a problem might seem good at the time but could have terrible consequences. My second book, *The Cloned Identity,* has also been published. Both these books were written some thirty years ago, but the contents are very up to date. I seem able to look years ahead and see what could or will probably happen in the future. As they say, I am not always right, but I am never wrong.

It is very sad when couples split with anger and despair as the children will suffer more than the parents. The same result follows when both parents try to prove they are the best parent and the other is the faulty one and should be the blamed one. There could be a thousand reasons to hate someone, and thousands of festering minutes you could spend in your life trying to convince yourself or others, but you can never change your history. The minute you can change is now; your history is embedded for all your life. You can live every second in the past and spend every second in misery, or you can move on and live in happiness. That choice is yours and no one else's.

If you are asked to write a four-letter word and you write 'HATE' instead of 'LOVE', you would cry instead of smile; yet you really know what the best is for you. You can never hate someone more than you can hate yourself, and you can never blame someone more than you can blame yourself; but you can hurt others more than you can hurt yourself.

CHAPTER NINE

HISTORY IN THE MAKING

This chapter was originally written for the benefit of my brothers, who were too young to understand the complexity of what went on in life round them during their early childhood. I hope it answers some of the questions they may have wondered about as they became older, and it may help to explain why their lives and mine have been so different.

The furthest back I can remember is when I was aged about three years and living at the Coles bakery at Sandringham Drive just off the Narborough road. In those days both Mum and Dad worked during the day and Gran would look after Terry and me. Most of the information I have from this time was given to me by Gran.

Gran said that although Terry was older I grew bigger and stronger and was far more inquisitive. I always wanted to know and wanted to do. Terry would always do as he was told and behave correctly, whereas I was always into something. But at the same time Terry was always there for me, and it was very traumatic for me when one day he never came home from school. He disappeared from my life for ever. Gran told me that when he was at school I would spend the day out and about the bakery site and I would give her kittens when she went out to find me. She would find me in the orchard, the workshops, the garage or the bakery, under a van or the bakery machinery.

Mum would sometimes in the summer be working at the lido near Leicester. She was in charge of the catering, so Terry and I would go with her and Gran would come to look after us while Mum worked. Gran told me that Terry would stay with her, but I would always be off finding out what was going on. On many occasions I gave her kittens because I used to waddle when walking and I would stray very close to the edge of the pool, but I never fell in.

In my whole life I have never eaten a mince pie or anything containing mincemeat. The reason I have put down to an incident Gran once told me.

One day I was in the kitchen having tea and Mum came in and, as usual, asked me what I had been doing that day.

I blurted out, "Been in bakery squirting shit into them cakes."

Although Mum and Gran could not stop laughing, Gran told me later that Mum went mad at the bakers for telling me what to say. It seemed as though the men in the bakery were always telling me what to say. They would also stand me on a stool at one of the machines where the mince pies were made and show me how to pull the lever to squirt the mincemeat into the pastry cups.

I grew up very quickly. Gran told me that when they took me for my first day at school many of the other kids were crying and had to be dragged into school by the teachers, but when they came for me I shrugged off their hands and just ran into the school. I never even looked back. That was upsetting for both Gran and Mum. It must have brought back memories of when they brought Terry to school.

This part is very emotional for me and very difficult for me to put into words.

When Terry came home from school he came on the bus which used to set off from Narborough and went to Enderby past what was called the looney bin. This was an asylum for dangerous persons. They would sound the siren if someone escaped. When we went and looked through the railings we could see some of them walking about. They didn't look dangerous, but we would run if they walked towards us. The school kids got on the bus outside the Co-op in Enderby. The bus travelled down to the roundabout, turned right and went along the Narborough road back to the start. It would stop by Mrs Druce's house, opposite Sandringham Drive, and Mum would be waiting, talking to the other women. Terry would get off, and when the bus had left and the women had finished their chat Mum would cross the road with Terry and walk up the road to home. That was the normal routine.

However, one fatal day Dad had a big job on at the bakery and he asked Mum to do something for him. As a result Mum wasn't at the bus stop to meet Terry. This would not normally have been a problem because the other women, especially Mrs Druce, would be there to look after Terry. But when Terry got off the bus and couldn't see Mum waiting he probably thought he would run up the lane and meet her. The road was a dual carriageway with a central reservation with tall hedges, taller than a child, so the lorry on its way to Leicester would not have seen Terry crossing and Terry would not have seen the lorry; so the one-in-a-million chance happened.

That day changed my life, and Gran told me how it changed Mum and Dad's life for evermore. Mum and Dad's first reaction was quite normal: they were both together and consoled each other for the grief they both felt, but after the funeral Gran said there was a complete change in both of them. Mum blamed herself and she blamed Dad because she had not been there to meet the bus. Dad blamed only himself. From that moment on there was a rift between them for the rest of their life. Even when Mum knew she was dying she would have nothing to do with Dad.

During the time I spent with Mum at Rowcroft, the local hospice, she poured out a lot of her life and was so very bitter about so much. It was a pity she wasn't able to talk to Dad because they both suffered the same grief, and it bothered me. It made me realise how important reconciliation is to life in general, and I have been very moved by the statue of *Reconciliation* in Coventry Cathedral.

Mum was constantly having a go at Dad, and he could never do anything right. I believe that the circumstances of Terry's death explain why that was.

My life without Terry was a different one. Gran told me that for days after he was killed I would, as before, wait by the gate at the same time, expecting to see him coming home from school. I was too young to understand what being dead actually meant.

In one of the houses opposite the bakery there was a family, and Mum arranged for their daughter Sandra, who was older and at school (she was aged seven or eight) to come and play with me when she wasn't at school. Gran told me that, being a typical girl, she enjoyed teasing me, which was a silly thing to do.

I had a pedal car (a Jeep) and a tricycle. Gran said she remembered sitting on the house step having a cup of tea when she saw me suddenly stop in the Jeep, stand on the seat, beat my chest with my hands and roar. Sandra laughed at me, so I ran at her, dragged her off the bike, lifted her above my head and threw her over my Jeep. She ended up in a crumpled heap. Gran had to look after her and console her with some sweets as she didn't want Sandra looking upset when her mother came to collect her.

Even at that age I had well above the normal strength and power. When I was in the workshops with Fred Martin he was always surprised at what I could carry.

The owner of the bakery lived in the big house and offices at the other side of the site to our house. He had a wife or daughter called Gwen. She had a car and on a Friday would take the wages to the bread shops over quite a large area. Sometimes she would take me. Because when I sat in the passenger seat I couldn't see over the dashboard I used to stand up to see the road ahead. Whenever she used the brakes I would bang my head on the windscreen and she would tell me to sit down. I would do so for a couple of seconds, then I was up again – so even at that age I had plenty of bangs on my head, but not nearly as bad as in 2005 when a scaffold pole smashed the side of my head.

One day I caused quite a panic. If Mum was off working in Leicester and Gran wasn't there, Dad would drop me and my pedal car in Enderby village at Lexie's. Lexie and George were long-time friends of Mum and Dad. They lived in a prefab and I spent a lot of time there. But this day was different for some reason. Lexie had some other women round for a cup of tea and chat, and when they left she realised I was not there. She panicked and ran everywhere, but I could not be found. That started a mass panic in Enderby. Soon everybody in the village was looking for me. Lexie rang my dad at work, and he came in the van and searched Enderby, but there was still no sign of me. As a last resort he drove along the bus route back to Sandringham Drive. He saw my Jeep parked by the wall of a house on the Narborough road, and, looking over the wall, he saw me sitting by a pond full of goldfish. I was probably aged three or four, not yet at school, and Stewart was not yet born, yet I had pedalled across Enderby and down the main road, then along the Narborough road (probably a distance of four miles), then climbed over a wall – a feat that was the talk of Enderby for some time. Today, when I look at children of that age, I realise just how far ahead of my age I was.

By the time Stewart was born Mum had been working for some time. With the grief she felt regarding Terry she had no interest in Stewart, and as a result Stewart was looked after by Gran, me and Dad. I spent a lot of time with Gran, and I believe none of us looked on Stewart as a Terry replacement. Nobody would ever be accepted as that. Gran called him the wanderer as he was always on his own. Perhaps it was unfortunate that he was born so close to Terry's death; but although he didn't receive a lot of love and attention from Mum, he was treated normally by everyone else. Lexie was more of a mother to him than his real mother was.

When the twins were born we had moved to 66 Trinity Road. When we first moved there it was a new housing estate, and our number was not 66 at first. The council made a mistake and had to renumber the houses. It was quite an exciting time having a brand-new house with four bedrooms and a nice garden. Also there were plenty of other families with children and we all enjoyed a good childhood there.

I remember when Peter nearly lost his finger when Paul closed a drain cover. What was Peter doing with his hand down a drain? I believe I could identify the exact drain cover if it is still there. I could even re-enact that moment, I remember it so vividly. Paul just did what he was told by an adult. Peter died in 2011, at the age of sixty, and we all miss him.

When we first moved to Trinity Road the twins were still in their pram. It was a big black Silver Cross pram and they would sit looking at each other. Stewart would climb up on the wheels and whack whichever one was crying or yelling then whack the other. Gran or I would have to get him down. He could climb up but couldn't get himself down, so sometimes we would find him sitting with the twins or even lying asleep with them in the pram.

One Boxing Day Mum decided we should go and spend the day with Gran in Leicester. The problem was that there were no buses on Boxing Day. Mum, being Mum, wasn't going to be put off, so we set out to walk there. We had the twins and Stewart in the pram and I walked with Mum and Dad. I had just started school so was about six. It was a very long walk (probably eight to ten miles), freezing cold and there was snow on the ground. We started about 8 a.m. and got there about 3 p.m. Gran had a small house with an outside loo, no lighting and a small open fire. I don't think I ever got warm again during our visit, but it was a good trip for the twins and Stewart, who kept warm and cosy in the pram. Next day we returned home by bus.

In Enderby after school I would get on the bus and it would travel almost the same route as Terry's bus, except that it would turn left at the roundabout and go in the opposite direction, towards Leicester. Our bus stop was opposite the estate, and all the mothers would be there to meet us and see us across the road. Some of us would spend our penny bus fare in a little shop in Enderby. We would then have to run across the fields to beat the bus to the bus stop. We would then hide behind the hedge till the bus stopped, and when the other kids got off we would pop over so it seemed as though we had come on the bus. I don't think we were ever caught out, but sometimes we had to run the mile and a half like the wind. Was the penny lolly worth it? I am not so sure, looking back, but it seemed fun at the time.

While I was at Enderby Primary School for the harvest festival or at Easter the pupils and staff would walk the short distance to the church and listen to a sermon by the vicar. I would enjoy the singing – 'We Plough the Fields and Scatter', etc. – but would find the other parts of the service boring and would spend the time staring at the golden-eagle lectern. I have never forgotten the golden eagle. Sitting in the church, I would be aware that Terry was buried quite close. This was my secret from the other kids, and I probably used the eagle as a way of keeping to myself the grief I always felt while sitting in the church.

When I was aged three or four, I was often asked to act as a pageboy dressed in frilly shirts and satin trousers. I think Mum used to hire me out. The main reason was because I had curly hair. My nickname was Bubbles, and I was to find out later that this was taken from a picture reproduced in the *Pear's Cyclopaedia* which showed a picture of a little boy blowing bubbles; the boy had curly hair the same as mine. To keep my hair in order Mum would take me to the barber's in Enderby and give him specific instructions on how to cut it and taper the curls.

While at Trinity Road we only ever once went to Leicester to meet Dad's father. After that we never saw him again. Apparently Dad's mother had died – I don't know when or why – but then his father married again but did not tell Dad or Ron. He just turned up one day with his new pregnant wife. That upset Dad more than Ron – so much so that he would not have anything more to do with him. Ron tried to mend the rift on many occasions, but to no avail. If Ron was in Leicester, he would come to see us and he would bring Jimmy, who was a stepbrother to Dad. But, despite Ron's trying, Dad would have nothing to do with Jimmy or his father.

I can remember many arguments between Dad and Ron over that, but at least Ron kept coming to see us. If he was working close to where we were living, he would stay with us. That happened in Southall and Kenton. Although Ron was invited to all our weddings he never came to all of them. That was because of the way Dad had been with his father and Jimmy. Ron never married, despite being quite a good catch for the ladies. I think the way Mum and Dad behaved put him off completely. I knew that when he was there Mum would be having a go at Dad over some silly thing. It didn't bother Dad – he was used to it – but it used to make Ron feel uncomfortable and he would go and sit in his room. I would sometimes join him and we would talk quite a lot. I always thought Ron had a lot of sense. He made time for people, and he made the best of his life, but his main direction was diverted by his father's and our father's stupidity. I feel you have to be able to accept that everybody is different, and everybody is entitled to a life and entitled to live it the way that suits them. Nobody has the right to force others to change their way.

Dad and Ron were both called up for the Second World War, but they were not allowed to join the forces as they were both considered too useful with their engineering experience. Only Norman was sent to fight, yet the work Dad and Ron were doing was more dangerous in some ways than fighting in the trenches. Their job was in the Midlands, where the factories were constantly being bombed by the Germans during the night. As soon as the all-clear sounded, in some cases before gangs of men went into the bombed factories, their job was to salvage any equipment they could find, transport it to another location and get it working again. Their job was very dangerous owing to unexploded and time-delayed bombs still lying in the buildings. Quite often the Germans would send some more bombers, which would turn up from a different direction to attack the emergency services. Dad told me he lost quite a good few men in this way. A tremendous number of people – many of them civilians – lost their lives in these air raids, and sometimes their bodies were never found. Dad was annoyed at times because London seemed to be the only city referred to when the media highlighted the air raids, yet more damage was done to the cities of the Midlands because that was where most of the factories and industry vital to the war was situated.

Also in the Midlands there were some American bases, which Dad used to visit on the scrounge. The Americans had so much more in the way of equipment than we did. Dad said they were so supportive to us and would let us have any surplus they had – even transport. Tools like jacks and winches were especially useful. One of the bases was set up for the invasion, and thousands of lorries, Jeeps, etc. were camouflaged over fields as far as you could see. The American engineers had built a garage-type inspection pit, which was about a mile long, and vehicles were over the pit so the engineers could work on the vehicles like an assembly line. Occasionally Dad would return to Leicester with food and other items given by the Yanks, but because no one had any money he could not make any money from what he had. All he could do was to exchange them for other things. As he said, there were a lot of people who had nothing but the clothes on their backs so he was happy to give and help if he could. Just after the war he said he could have bought a house for £5, but no one had £5. You would have to go without – even starve for a couple of years or more – to get £5. People were having to sleep rough in makeshift tents and forage round for food just to exist. They had nowhere else to live.

The factories had been bombed, and the ones which had been able to carry on were involved only with the war effort. Many industries were closed down and workers found themselves out of a job. Dad and Ron were lucky in that respect as the bakery industry was still important and needed engineers to maintain the equipment.

When Norman came home he and Margret stayed with Mum and Dad and Gran. All Norman had was his uniform; he was given no money for the time he spent in the army – not like today. He told me that when they got back to the base it was not like returning home; within twenty-four hours they were demobbed, given a rail warrant and sent home. They received no thanks. They just said goodbye to any mates they still had left and went out into the wilderness. Many of them had no home or job to return to. At times, like most of those who came back, he wasn't sure who exactly won the war. They, the so-called winners, were worse off than if they had not gone to war. For some, even if the Germans had won they could hardly have been worse off than they were.

I can see that both Mum and Dad had miserable lives. Why? Perhaps they could not come to terms with the blame they put on themselves. Mum covered that up by putting Dad down all the time; and her attitude made it hard for Dad to accept his responsibility and work out an amicable solution. Because neither could accept that life could be better they both, in my opinion, wasted what could have been an amazing happy life. Instead they both spent it in what I call the room of solace.

What I am writing does not always flow in the correct time sequence, but that is because it seems appropriate to record my memories in the sequence they come to my mind.

There is, however, one event which I have put off recording. I have found it too traumatic to write about it before. On the day of Terry's funeral I spent the day at Mrs Druce's house, and Gran told me that in the evening she, Dad and Mum collected me and we all went up to the church at Enderby and stood by Terry's grave. We stayed there for a long emotional time.

As we were leaving, Mum said to me, "Say goodnight to Terry, David."

I shouted out, "I can't. He's dead."

That broke all their hearts. It was a very emotional moment for us all. That memory has always been with me, and for me to write it still brings tears to my eyes. It will take a while before I calm down.

Gran told me that event many, many times. I was only three years old, but I must have overheard the adults talking about it before the funeral. I believe that moment was a turning point in our lives, and what I said brought home to Mum and Dad the reality that Terry had gone. Gran said after that day they seemed very different people towards each other, and they never visited Terry's grave together again for a very long time. Even then they didn't show their emotions together and never talked about Terry between themselves.

I spent a lot of time with Mrs Druce. I think she never stopped blaming herself for letting Terry run across the road, and looking after me was a way to repay Mum. She taught me how to sew and knit, and at Enderby School, despite being a boy, I was the best at sewing and knitting – far better than any of the girls. This often bemused the teachers. When I finally got to the last year, in Bob West's classes I was always best at craft. He used me to help the others. It was then I realised that some just could not do the things I found so easy.

In one lesson Mr West wanted to teach us how to use a pen. (In those days we used a dip pen with a metal nib.) He sat at a desk and wrote his name and address; then, with his arms folded, and in his usual shouting voice, he told us to do the same. We then had to take our writing to him so that he could compare our efforts with his and laugh at our attempts. He enjoyed belittling the pupils, and he called some idiots and worse. He was quite enjoying himself until I took mine to show him and he could see that my writing was better than his – not that he would say that. He just jumped up and started on another lesson. He never did a writing lesson like that again. By today's standard he would be considered a bully.

In those days the teachers at primary schools were mainly women, but every primary school had a man teacher and he always seemed to have an elevated position. He was like a father figure. The head teacher at Enderby was Lily Clark, but even she seemed to look up to Mr West – OK, she was only half his height and he would tower over her. I had my knuckles rapped by the edge of her ruler on many occasions – usually because I was helping others. The pain didn't stop me smiling at her no matter how hard she hit my knuckles. I knew I was right and they were wrong.

I was told much later that Lily Clark and the other staff had been very supportive to Mum and Dad when Terry died. He had been a well-liked pupil at the school.

Just before I started school I used to go with Dad when he had to go to see the local policeman with the bakery vehicles' paperwork. The policeman's name was Taylor and he was a nice man. We would go to his police house and he and Dad would sit and have a cup of tea in the kitchen while they went through the paperwork. He would stand on a chair and reach down his revolver from on top of the cupboard and let me play with it. I was aged only four at the time. By the time I started school I already knew the workings of a Webley 45-calibre revolver and how to swing a truncheon.

Before long Coles sold the bakery to Elkes of Uttoxeter and they started building everywhere. The land that was next to our house, which was the tennis courts, was used to build a new factory unit to produce chocolate products. Dad brought a block of chocolate in one day, but it was horrible – not like sweet chocolate – so I was disappointed. They then decided they needed our house for offices, so we were moved to a much smaller house on the edge of Enderby village. This did at least back on to the Enderby recreational park so we had a nice playground as a garden.

Two doors up was the police house. PC Taylor had gone from Narborough and we now had a new village policeman. His name was Dixon; and whereas everyone liked Taylor, who mixed and was friendly with everyone, nobody liked Dixon, who was a totally by-the-book policeman and was never friendly with anyone. The only time he ever went into the Nag's Head was to nick someone for some trivial infringement.

His son was at our school, and he was treated favourably by Mr West because of who his father was. He wasn't very well liked by the other boys for the same reason. One time one of the boys whacked him and he shouted out that his father would stop our bus, which went past his house, and drag us off and lock us all up. We were all frightened when the bus approached the Dixon house, but, much to our relief, the bus was not stopped. We were feeling quite chuffed until someone said he was probably waiting at our bus stop, so we were all looking out with apprehension as the bus stopped at our stop. We lived to fight another day, but not before we had all spent a worried evening at home expecting a knock on the door.

We spent just over a year in this small house. I could easily walk to school from there, and there were always plenty of children in the rec.

Then we got our new house at Trinity Road, which had a big kitchen and four bedrooms. Stewart and I had our own bedrooms. In the back of the fireplace in the back living room was an oven accessible from the kitchen. We also had a front room, which we hardly ever used.

Because of Dad's job we were the only house to have a telephone, and I can remember so many times having to run and fetch a neighbour because the call was for them. Neighbours also used to pop in to make a call and always left the money (usually a few pennies).

Because we had a front room Mum decided I would play the piano; so Dad had to find and buy a piano. He got it in the neck when that turned up because Mum had it in her head it should be a baby grand and it was just a small upright pub-type piano. But Dad pointed out that a baby grand was not only too expensive but would not fit in the house let alone fit in the front room. Mum then got me music lessons from Margret's father, so I had to get a bus into Leicester and walk to his house to learn the piano. This turned into a disaster because I was not musical and never would be. I am more of a drum player, if anything. Margret's father wrote a letter to Mum explaining that it was a waste of time. Mum went through the roof, as usual, and I was blamed for not trying. Dad was blamed for buying the wrong piano; then he was blamed for not being in charge of me and not making me practise. I ended up with my trousers down across the pouffe, and I got the leather belt across the bottom with all Dad's might. I ended up in pain and crying, whereon Mum felt sorry for me and blamed Dad for hurting me.

Yes, many times I received a good hiding from Dad so he could keep Mum happy, yet she always regretted causing it. How come I was the only one who got the beating? At times I would be beaten for protecting one of my brothers, but I don't remember any of them ever doing that for me.

In wintertimes we spent a lot of time sitting in front of the fire, and Mum would tell us a story which she invented. Some were quite nasty.

Chickens have just come to mind. When we lived at the bakery site there was a large orchard with hundreds of chickens. They were there for the eggs the bakery required. There were no supermarkets in those days and most families used dried egg, but at the bakery we had the real thing. If Norman and Margret came for the weekend, and if Mr Coles was away, I would go with Dad and Norman into the orchard and we would catch a couple of the chickens. Norman would wring their necks, and we would then take them into the workshop and pluck them. Norman would then place some of the chicken parts we didn't need by the fence in the orchard so it would look as though a fox had got them. I was probably the only three-year-old chicken-plucker in Leicester. I found the feathers went up my nose and made me have a sneezing fit.

When we lived at Trinity Road Mum used to work at the Granby at various functions. The ones I remember most clearly were the Jewish ones because she always brought home a bag of chicken – kosher chicken, to be exact. We lived on kosher chicken for a few days – not that we would know the difference between kosher and non-kosher. Chicken was very expensive because the farmers concentrated on producing eggs for the food industry rather than meat.

When she was working on Saturday night at the Granby Mum did not get home till the early hours on Sunday, so she would stay in bed till lunchtime. Sunday breakfast was cooked by Dad, and it was always bacon, egg, tomatoes and fried bread. This became known as 'the Hughes breakfast'. I helped to get lunch ready by getting the vegetables from the garden. My brothers would never eat their sprouts or cabbage so I always had plenty of vegetables to eat.

Many years later, working in the food industry, I was to realise just how important it is to grow your own vegetables and eat fresh. Most of the vegetables we bought in the shops were grown in Norfolk and sent to Covent Garden Market in London. Then they would be sold and transported to shops around the country. To keep them as fresh as possible, when the vegetables were harvested they would be dipped in ethylene glycol. This, as you may know, is actually used for antifreeze in vehicles.

Back at the bakery one of the men I remember most clearly is Fred Martin. He was a sort of general worker. He did carpentry, etc., and he also used to set the traps to catch the rats. I used to spend time in his workshop, and he would show me the cage with the rat in. Outside he had an old water drum he used to put the cage in for a while; then he would lift it out and show me the result. I always remember his words: "Dead rat!" He lived in Enderby and some Sunday afternoons we would walk up to visit him and his wife. He was a good gardener and I used to explore his sheds while the adults had tea and cakes.

Mum decided I would be a choirboy, which meant in the dark and wet I would cycle along the pavement to Narborough Church. Mum had decided I would be the top choirboy, but the choirmaster told me I was tone deaf and wouldn't be any use as a choirboy. He told Mum, but I still got the blame and another hiding. It's good being the eldest, don't you think?

When we moved to Southall I went to Featherstone Primary School, which I found in some ways better then Enderby. It was larger and better equipped. But living in Southall was a complete change from Enderby, where we had been a smaller close-knit community in a country environment. Our new town environment took a lot of getting used to, but I found it better for learning and growing up.

I soon became top in the JTC section of the Church Lads' Brigade, and when we went to summer camp in Dorset, back in my country environment, I had a lot of advantages over the town boys and would win most (if not all) of the competitions. When we paraded in the hall we would be inspected by the officer, and the boy who had the best turnout was called the 'stickman'. I would always be the 'stickman' until one evening one of the officers, Mr Fletcher (he later went on to be a vicar), called me to one side and told me that I would not be 'stickman' for a while. I accepted what he said, but didn't ask why. I later found out the reason was that some of the parents had complained: their boys were disheartened when I always won, so they would never bother. My opinion is that they should have tried harder and not given up. From then on whenever the one who won looked at me with a happy smirk it never bothered me because I knew the reason he had won.

I expect my brothers do not have many recollections about Southall because they were very young at the time. John was born in the big flat we had in King Street above Harrington's bakery shop, and I can still remember that evening well. I recall the shouting from the midwife to Dad to bring hot water.

I also remember John's christening at St John's by the Reverend Morley. I thought he was the best vicar ever. I spent many good hours helping him with printing, and I actually printed the form for John's christening. We stood in the church as Mr Morley gave his sermon, and John, having gone a whole twenty minutes without being fed, started yelling and drowned the sermon. Mr Morley stopped and asked Mum to go outside and do what was necessary to quieten him down. Mum wasn't very happy at being told what to do, but she carried out the instructions so when John was dipped in the font everyone was happy, including him.

When we had the fire in the kitchen of the flat Mr Morley was there within minutes offering help and support, and the Church sent crockery and cutlery, etc. It was a big fire, probably caused when Mum left the grill on – but the cause of the fire was not disclosed, as I remember. The flat was uninhabitable, so Mum and my brothers were taken in by the couple who lived in the flat above the Bata shoe shop. They were the managers there. They did not have any children of their own, but one of them might have been one of John's godparents (I'm not sure). They had become good friends of us all. Because they had limited space Dad and I bedded down in the burnt-out flat. I can still remember the smell of the fire. Harrington's was very supportive and we were quickly moved into another flat at Kenton.

Kenton was another complete change of direction for us. It was also when I started my cycling career. When we moved to Kenton I still stayed at Featherstone County Secondary Boys' School. Later I was glad I did. It was entirely my decision. Dad had arranged for me to change school because of the travelling, but Mum supported me, saying that it would be easier for me to go to the same school as Stewart, etc. It was a short walk to Kenton Station, and from there I was able to take the train, but at first I travelled to Southall by bus (I caught the number 140 bus to the Grapes at Hayes, then the trolleybus along the Uxbridge Road to Southall Broadway, then the number 105 bus to near the school).

Harrington's gave Dad a Morris van to go to work in, but I usually had to leave before him. When he left early he would give me a lift to the Grapes public house on the Uxbridge Road. It would have been quite easy for him to drop me at the school, like many parents do these days, but no matter how bad the weather was he would only drop me at the Grapes. In good weather I would cycle to and from school.

I used to do odd little jobs to earn money so I could get myself a racing bike, and I eventually managed to buy a Claud Butler. I found out later that Claud Butler was arrested and prosecuted; he could not produce enough bike frames himself, so he bought in from other manufacturers and changed the name to his own – so my bicycle might not have been the genuine article. I covered thousands of miles, including cycling to school, and would sometimes just go off for a couple of weeks. I don't think Mum and Dad ever really knew where I was, although I was only twelve or thirteen, and neither took any interest.

I was in several cycling clubs. I worked every Saturday, and on Sunday I would usually cycle fifty to eighty miles. Dad arranged a holiday at Hayling Island, and as his van wasn't very big and there was Mum, Dad, Peter, Paul, Stewart, John and Gran he asked if I could cycle there. I got the impression he expected me to do that anyway. So on that day I set off early and got to Guildford before he overtook me. He pipped his horn and just drove by. I thought he would have stopped to check I was OK and say hello, but all I saw was the van go by and several little-brother faces peering out of the small back windows.

When I finally reached Hayling, there was a problem because the van and Dad were not there – just Gran and my brothers. Gran told me Mum had been taken to hospital with a problem; so it was good that Gran was there, but it wasn't much of a holiday for her. She did the cooking, and I helped her with my brothers. Mum was in hospital for several days and spent only a couple of days at the holiday home before the trip home.

I wonder if my brothers ever go up Porlock Hill, and if it reminds them of the brother who rode up it on his bike. Come to think of it, none of them ever travelled by pushbike in their lives.

At Kenton a few doors from us lived a family who ran a fish-and-chip shop. Mum got a job there in the evenings and on Saturdays, and I would help out at times. Then the man became often ill, so I helped him and he taught me how to prepare the fish and batter. He became too ill to work, and after he died I used to help his wife. Often she would forget to order the fish, so I would cycle with a bucket to get supplies from a fish shop at Wealdstone. It was a bit difficult riding a bike holding a bucket of fish.

Mum used to get me plenty of other jobs from the customers. I was always cleaning cars, digging gardens, etc., etc.

The couple who owned the shop used to always go down to Worthing on the early closing day, Wednesday, and one time they took Mum, Stewart and me. Peter and Paul were left with Gran. They also took us into a café in Worthing for a meal. Stewart upset Mum because he wanted the most expensive item on the menu, which was a mixed grill; then – typical Stewart! – he left most of it. He had never had it before, and he didn't like it. That was the first time we had been to that part of the coast.

I also remember the Easter holidays we had at Skegness and Yarmouth and the times when Mum and Dad had to sit at each end of the caravan to stop it blowing over in the hurricane storms. It took all day to get there from Leicester in our Austin 7, and on one occasion a spring broke on the way back and we all had to sit on one side to balance the car so we could get home.

One of the cycle rides I did was from Kenton to Portsmouth. I then took the ferry across to the Isle of Wight. The youth hostel was full at Cowes, so I booked the following night and went back to a youth hostel in the New Forest. The next day I returned to the Isle of Wight and spent the day there.

While coming down a hill a bee flew into my shirt, and by the time I stopped and pulled it out it had stung my chest. I was in agony; so I went into a chemist, and the lady in there put something on the sting and used tweezers to pull the barb out.

I spent the night at the youth hostel at Cowes, which was an amazing place with views across the valley. It's a crying shame that none of my brothers experienced youth hostelling. It was an amazing experience. Next day I cycled to Yarmouth, caught the ferry back to the mainland and cycled along the coast to my next youth hostel at Bridport. In my CLB days we had camped at Corfe Castle and Bridport, so I knew much of Dorset. I always thought I would live in Dorset one day. Who knows!

Next day I went on to Lyme Regis. It was great freewheeling down the hill into Lyme, but not so good at the bottom when I realised I had to go back up! Then I came inland to Marlborough and turned east on to the A4 to make my way back to London and home. It had taken me two weeks to do that trip.

On another trip from Kenton, I met up with a friend from school, Alf Kennedy. Later I was his best man when he married Sue. His parents, sister and two uncles were into horse racing and would often have a holiday at Newton Abbot during the racing season. They asked me to visit them, so I left Kenton very early and cycled to Newton Abbot – over 200 miles. It was two o'clock in the morning when I got to the top of Telegraph Hill. It was pitch-black and I couldn't see the road, so it was quite a difficult ride.

When I reached Newton Abbot I decided to look for somewhere to sleep. I didn't know there was a train station in Newton Abbot, so I cycled to the train station in Teignmouth and the guard let me sleep in the waiting room as long as I left before the inspector came round in the morning.

I spent two days with the Kennedys then cycled back to Kenton. My brothers later travelled the road from London to Torquay; I wonder if they gave some thought to the fourteen-year-old who cycled that route on his own.

Other destinations of mine included the Brecon Beacons in Wales,

Southend, Oxford, Aylesbury, Box Hill and Bristol.

At one of the cycling clubs we had a man called David Handley. He was training for the World Championships at Leipzig, where he actually won a bronze medal, so he was the third best sprinter in the world at that time. On two of his training sessions with us I was able to outsprint him; and his manager, Bob Gale, said he would like to train me when I was old enough to enter the Olympics. This would have cost me a lot of money and time, and I would have had to obtain some sponsorship. There was no way I could do that or ask my parents to raise the money. When Bob Gale came home from the championships he showed me the bronze medal and said, "You would have had silver." This was just a pipe dream for a fourteen-year-old as any thought of being in the Olympics seemed a million years away.

When I moved from bikes to a scooter I had to split the bike and sell it as bits as no one had the money to afford the complete bike. Mum and Dad (who supported Mum to keep the peace) said I wasn't to buy a motorbike, so (to keep the peace too) I bought an old Lambretta 125 for £10. I had to do some repairs to it, but I managed to ride it to Bristol one Christmas. There was a lot of snow and ice and I became very cold. At Bristol I sat in front of a roaring fire, but couldn't feel warm for hours.

I then bought a larger scooter – a DKR Cappella. It had a 150cc Villiers engine, but that was not powerful enough so I looked around a scrapyard in London near the *Cutty Sark* and found a 250cc twin Villiers motorbike engine. I wrote to the makers of DKR at Wolverhampton and asked them for advice, and they took some months to send me a letter saying it was impossible to fit the 250cc engine in my frame. By that time I was able to write back and tell them I had fitted it and was using it. To fit the engine I had to cut and weld alterations to the frame; design, make and fit new engine mounts; design, make and fit a new wiring loom; design and weld a new twin-exhaust system; and design and fit an air-flow system to stop the covered engine from overheating. During the summer months I would have to leave the side panels off to increase the cooling. The biggest problem I had was with the gearing. Because of the design of the rear wheel I could not fit a smaller-diameter sprocket, which meant

I would get wheel spin when I tried to pull away in top gear, so I could get through a lot of back tyres if I used too much power.

Ray Warner, the best man at my wedding, bought the scooter off me when I moved on to cars.

When we lived at Wembley Mum decided we needed another front room, so builders were summoned to convert the garage into a room. Why a front room when another bedroom would be of more use? The front room was hardly ever used. I used to play my records, and I was not impressed when Stewart played them when I wasn't around. I didn't mind him playing them, but I kept them tidy and in their correct sleeves (I still have them just like that), whereas Stewart just chucked them around and some became scratched. I was soon to learn more about Stewart's ways.

One day we couldn't get in the bathroom, so I stood on a chair and looked through the window. I could see Stewart lying on the floor, so I forced the door open and checked he was still breathing. He was, but we couldn't get him to wake up, so Mum and I managed to get him to bed and I kept an eye on him and flushed what was left of what he had been taking down the loo. He woke some hours later in another world. I can't remember exactly how many times I had to bring him back to the real world.

Stewart used to hang out at the Ace Café on the North Circular near Wembley. His nickname was the Duke. He never rode a motorbike, but was always smartly dressed so didn't look the biker part. He once bought a new pair of jeans and gave them to Mum with the instruction to wash and iron them. The washing was OK, but Mum didn't do much ironing. I always did my own. Well, when Stewart put the jeans on the creases were down the sides. Just imagine! He didn't see the funny side; he went mad and 'verbalised' Mum. Then he threw the jeans in the bin and stormed out. When I came home and found Mum in tears, and she told me why, I couldn't stop laughing. I got the jeans out of the bin, washed and ironed them properly and put them on his bed, but I found them in the bin again. I hope Stewart remembers that and laughs.

As I have related, when we moved to Bristol from Kenton it was arranged that I would go to Ashton Park, a coeducational school at Bedminster. A couple of years before, at Featherstone, a rumour had been going round that they were going to bring girls into the school and I can remember the words of the head, Mr Downs: "The day girls come in the front door I shall go out the back door."

Ashton Park was a big let-down for me. The teaching standard was not up to the quality of Featherstone, so moving to Bristol was not the best thing I did. The bakery Dad worked at was just round the corner, so he didn't have a van, and I couldn't see the point in moving to Bristol – especially as a few days after I left school Dad told me we were moving to Wembley.

When Gran came to stay with us in Bristol she was able to go through the backyard and be at the local pub in three minutes. Well, Gran came from Leicester, where they didn't drink much cider – she drank one glass of the local Kingston Black and was drunk. It took a few days for her to come to terms with that, but then she realised she could get merry with very little money.

When Norman and his family came for the weekend to pick Gran up she told him about the cider. Now, Norman was an eight-pints-of-mild-and-bitter man and didn't believe what she said, so Dad took Norman to the pub after tea to prove the point. Well, some time later we heard a commotion at the front door and opened it to find two very drunk men rolling about in the front garden. They then decided to set up a shop on the front doorstep, so emptied the larder of its contents and started selling like a market stall. We all left them to it and went to bed.

Next morning we found them snoring, fast asleep in the hall with the front door wide open. They had a bad head all day and got a lot of verbal from Mum and Margret. Norman never got over that: he had only two pints of what he thought tasted like lemonade and he was on his back. I don't think Dad or Norman drank cider ever again. Kingston Black is the only drink that ever brought Gran, Norman and Dad to their knees and gave them a headache.

At Bristol Mum had one of her usual brainwaves. She wanted a new kitchen, so she arranged for two carpenters from where she worked to come round and build it. After a few days they asked for payment for what they had done, and this sparked a big row between Mum and Dad because she had arranged it without asking him –

and not only that, but he didn't have the money. I had been doing eighteen-hour shifts at the bakery to cover men who were on holiday, so Dad asked me to lend him the money; so I did, but I never got it back. The two carpenters never turned up again, so when we later left Bristol the kitchen was still like a builder's yard.

Around the time of our move to Wembley was the time my brothers came of age in many ways and became more independent. Each one was different, but they were similar in many ways. Leicester, Southall, Kenton and Bristol were places they probably don't remember very much about, so they may not recall the amount of work Mum and Dad put into bringing up five boys on very little money – and never forget little Gran! She was beaten by her husband, Harry Aris, and yet was called a terrible women when she divorced him. Mum left home at sixteen because of the beating from her father, and her brother, Norman, was often beaten by his father when he tried to defend Gran and Mum. Nevertheless Gran was always there to help Mum and Dad by looking after us.

Mum used to drop me and Terry off at Gran's in Leicester when she went to work, and Gran would take us to Leicester Market, which was huge. When Mum picked us up she would ask Terry what we had done, and he would say, "Been to pub. One pint Vimto and crisps." Whenever Gran went to the market she would always pop into the pub for a drink and a chat with friends, and Terry and I would sit in the room at the back with our Vimto and crisps. Mum would always tell Gran off for taking us into the pub, but Gran never took any notice. It was probably the only bit of life she had. Gran told me about that, and she also told me that sometime after Terry's death she was talking to one of her friends when he pointed to me and said to Gran, "He's growling at me." Next thing he was hopping around yelling because I had sunk my teeth into his leg. Gran put it down to the fact that the man was standing where Terry used to stand, and I didn't want that. So I was a chicken-plucker at the age of three and a leg-biter at the age of four. What next?

When we lived at Wembley Mum decided to have a party at the Starlight Club. I think it was meant to be for her silver wedding, but

Gran told her she was wrong and her silver wedding was not for a couple of years. However, Mum took no notice of that fact, so the party took place with a lot of people invited, and it was quite a good evening. A few days later Dad got the bill, and as he just did not have that sort of spare money I gave him the money. He said he would pay me back, but I knew he never would.

Then Mum decided I would need a twenty-first birthday party and engagement party combined. As I have already related, this went ahead and was totally over the top: amazing food, waitresses and a toastmaster to myself. It all seemed so wrong, and I didn't have a very happy evening, but I went along with it because Mum was so happy. But again it cost much more than Dad could afford, so I paid for my own party.

One day Paul came home with some shrink-fit jeans. You had to put them on then spend a day soaking in the bath and let them dry while you were still wearing them so that they shrunk on your legs. That was OK if you had shapely legs, but Paul did look funny walking off down the road, displaying his spindly legs.

Another thing I associate with Paul is 'the morning after'. When Paul turned up at the breakfast table, I could tell by his facial expression whether or not he was in a bad mood. "Do not talk to me," his face seemed to say, but unfortunately Mum never detected this and she would go into her usual "What time did you get in? Where were you all night? Eat your breakfast. You won't be allowed out from this house without a full breakfast and you must wear your vest," etc., etc.

Paul would seem to listen carefully for the blink of an eye, then up he would jump, throw his breakfast across the table or on the floor and storm out. Mum would always look so surprised. She was probably thinking, 'Was it something I said?'

When I got married, Jennifer and her parents would have been more than happy with a simple wedding, but Mum didn't want that and she got her way. It was quite a big affair. Jennifer's parents just paid for some of the drink, and guess who paid the rest? Mum and Dad couldn't possibly have paid for it. And guess who paid for the weddings at Eastcote too, and where the money came from for the early caravans.

When I gave Dad my Vauxhall Magnum and I found out he had sold it he never asked if I wanted any of the money. And the control panel I designed, built and installed? Not a penny or even a 'thanks'! Dad would just ring up when he wanted a modification done; he never asked about the cost.

If Dad had been more in control and restrained Mum's ranting, things would have been much better for all of us. It seems to me that a lot of their troubles can be traced back to Terry's death. That is when things started to go wrong. If that hadn't happened, I believe we would have had a different upbringing, our whole lives would have been different, and we would have another brother – a brother I have missed so very much. I am having so many emotional storms as I write this. It's not easy when you can hardly see what you are typing through the tears falling down your face!

I've just thought about turkeys. When we were living at Trinity Road on Christmas Eve Dad and a lot of other men would go to Leicester Market because from about five o'clock in the evening of Christmas Eve the poultry traders would auction off any unsold turkeys. They had no cold stores, so you could bid and get a cheap buy. The longer you waited the cheaper they got – and also the bigger they were. One time Dad turned up with a turkey that was so big it wouldn't go in the oven, so Mum and Dad had to cut it into bits on the kitchen table. We lived on turkey for days.

Every day when Dad came home from work we would have fresh bread. He had an overcoat with poacher's pockets so he could put a loaf in each side and no one knew. Often there was also a bag of broken biscuits. So in the summer our tea was usually a doorstep of bread with real butter and plenty of home-made strawberry jam. I will always remember the three of us sitting at the table with our faces full of jam.

Rhubarb was another treat. Mum would make a cone of paper and put some sugar in, and we would have sticks of rhubarb to dip in and eat. In those days things were so simple. Just do a bit of scrumping and you had all the fresh and untarnished fruit you could eat! Who needed a supermarket!

A Mars Bar cost sixpence and was a very special treat, so we would slice it up to make it last longer. Spangles and Polos were also a treat. Fruit Salads and Blackjacks were four for a penny, so whenever we had a bottle to take back to the shop the penny deposit was useful. We quickly learnt the value of money and which sweets were the best buy for quantity and taste.

In those days no one seemed to have much money; everybody seemed to be in the same situation. Communities were like families so people knew one another, got on with one another, pooled together, helped one another, spoke to one another. Children grew up and played together. There were no computers, just clever, imaginative minds with a will to learn. We respected our elders. We could play all day in the fields. When we missed lunch we didn't go hungry; we ate an apple or a pear, plums or berries then just came home at teatime.

In the summer we used to play in the river, but that was stopped when an outbreak of polio was linked somehow to the river. At school in wintertime we were constantly told about coughs and sneezes spreading diseases, and to stop them by using our handkerchiefs.

School dinners were cooked by pupils' mothers and served by teachers. Produce was delivered to the school by local farmers, and everybody had a bottle of milk to start the day. It was good to be a milk monitor, to take the crates to each classroom, because there were always leftovers to drink.

Harvest time was a time to watch the steam engines and combine harvester at work, and the shotguns smoking as someone bagged a rabbit that had been running for its life.

We knew a policeman was a good friend, not an enemy. He was there to protect us from evil, and because of that he had our respect. If you made a silly mistake, you didn't get arrested and fined; you had a clip round the ear. And if you told your father, you got another clip and told not to do it again. In Leicester we would watch the policemen in awe in their smart uniforms and helmets, their smart capes hanging on the railings, directing the traffic round the clock tower with their white gloves.

The end? No, the beginning. Hopefully there are many more years to come.

CHAPTER TEN

PICTURE GALLERY

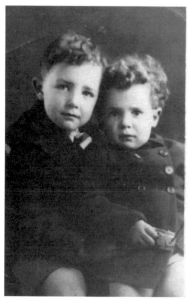

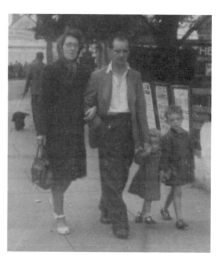

Mum and Dad.

Terry (b.1943) and David (b.1945)
Terry (1943–8).

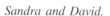

Sandra and David.

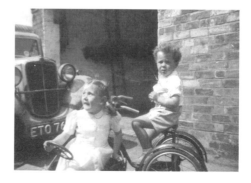

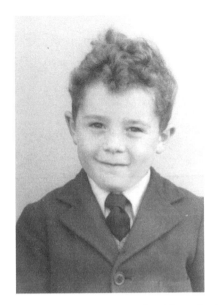
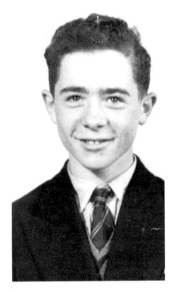

David – school photos.

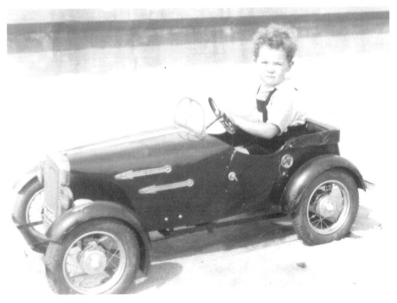

David learning to drive.

FEATHERSTONE COUNTY SECONDARY BOYS' SCHOOL
WESTERN ROAD, SOUTHALL

REPORT FOR YEAR ENDING JULY 1960

Name of pupil ... HUGHES David N.

Form ... 3 ... No. of pupils in form ... ... Position in form ... 1

SUBJECTS	% Marks obtained	*Assessment of years effort	REMARKS	Teacher's Initials
ENGLISH	65	B	A steady conscientious reader worker who has done well.	M B.
MATHEMATICS	48	B	Position 13th. A good year's work but examination result is very disappointing	CRN
SCIENCE CHEMISTRY	60	B	Good.	
PHYSICS	40	B	A good year's work.	
TECHNICAL DRAWING	50	C+	A real worker	
RELIGIOUS INSTRUCTION	74		Very good	K C M
GEOGRAPHY	80	A	Has found the way to make maximum progress	
HISTORY	48	C	4th in form. A satisfactory year's work	
ECONOMICS	63	B+	His work has been consistently at a high level. Well done!	MBF
FRENCH	60	B	Very satisfactory work	
ART & CRAFT	78	B	Always produces a neat & well finished exercise.	
WOODWORK	75	B.	Good work - keep it up	
METAL WORK	63	B	Fifth place in this subject. Well done	
PHYSICAL EDUCATION	79	B.	Very good result - hard worker	
MUSIC	59	C+	Quite a good effort.	

General Remarks :
Congratulations! You will need to work & work in your new form

He has made a conscientious effort in all subjects. A good, reliable worker, and an excellent result.

Conduct ... Excellent ... Progress ... Excellent

Times Absent ... 24 ... Times Late ... 2 ... (... Possible Attendances)

David's school report.

98

The

Church Lads' Brigade

JUNIOR TRAINING CORPS ATHLETE'S CERTIFICATE

This is to Certify that Junior *D M Hughes*

of *Sefton, Southall* Company, No. *3545* has passed the

INDIVIDUAL ABILITY TEST of the Junior Training Corps during the

year *1957* and is awarded his *1st* Class Certificate.

Date *4th Jan 1958*

General Secretary

NOTE.—The Test covered Sprinting, Long Distance Running, Jumping and Swimming

99

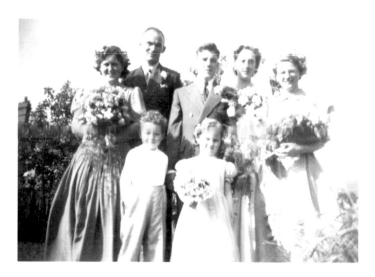

David the pageboy.

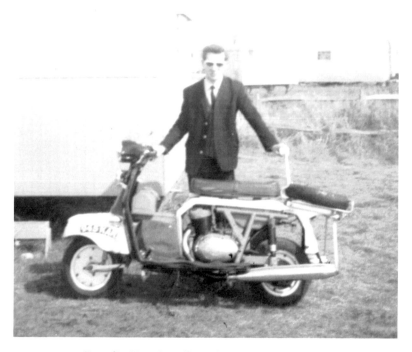

*David's CKR Capella with side panels removed
to cool the engine in summer, 1962—63.*

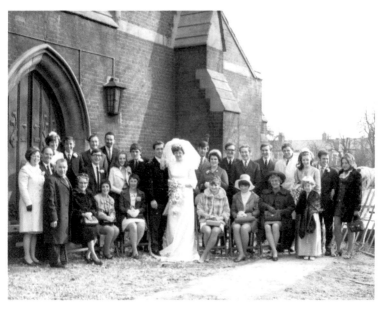

David's family on the occasion of his marriage to Jennifer,
St John's Church, Southall, Middlesex, 22 March 1969.

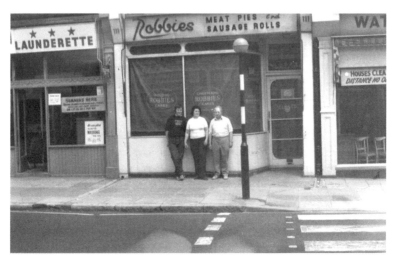

David's father, mother and brother John outside the bakery shop
in Southsea, 1975.

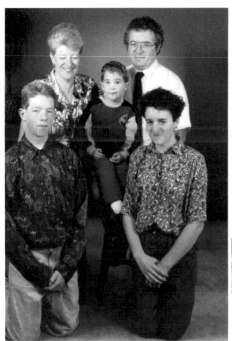

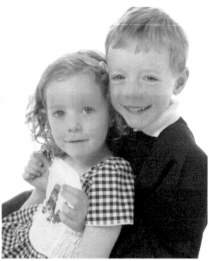

David's grandchildren,
Bethany and Joshua, 2010.

David's family, Gregory, Jennifer, Phillip,
David and Heidi, Torquay, 1990.

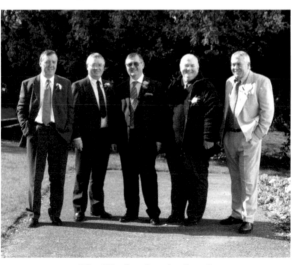

The Hughes brotherhood,
Paul, David, Peter, John and Stewart.

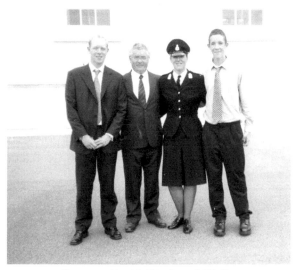

Gregory, David, Heidi and Phillip.
Heidi graduates from Sandhurst, 1999.

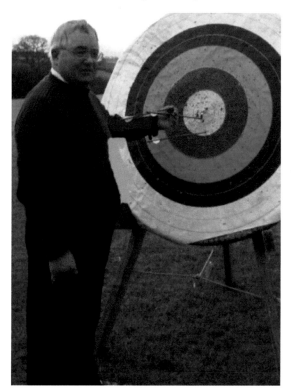

The first three arrows
twenty-five years on,
still on target,
Brixham Archery Club,
4 April 2012.

Details of Accident card which David carries to ensure that persons are aware
of his unusual medical condition and ensure he receives the correct assistance

FRONT of CARD

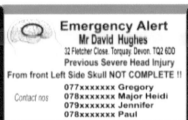

Emergency Alert
Mr David Hughes
32 Fletcher Close. Torquay. Devon. TQ2 6DD
Previous Severe Head Injury
From front Left Side Skull NOT COMPLETE !!

Contact nos
077xxxxxxx Gregory
078xxxxxxx Major Heidi
079xxxxxxx Jennifer
078xxxxxxx Paul

Back of CARD

Please Be Patience
David can become distressed agitated and
emotional upset he will take deep breaths
can hear but not able to speak or look this
can take 3-4 minutes to stabilise before
appearing calm and normal again

South Western Ambulance Service NHS
NHS Trust

Dear Mr Hughes,

Thank you for calling in to see me at Torquay Ambulance Station. I am always pleased to see people so that I can pass on their thanks to the crews involved in patient care, as this often gets missed. I am delighted that you have made such a fantastic recovery from the incident that took place on 4 August 2005.

We have now managed to trace the crews involved and three out of the four are still employed by the Trust and are in the process of sending on your gratitude to them for their professionalism and care to you as described in your letter. I was very interested in your description of the events that took place.

We have located the incident and the origin of the call was 10.53 am on the 4 August 2005. The crew arrived four minutes later at 10.57. Due to the seriousness of your condition they called for a second crew. The crew left scene at 11.36 after stabilising your condition and you arrived at Torbay Hospital at 11.41 am.

I hope this helps piecing together some of the events of the day in question and I hope that you continue to keep well for the future.

If I can be of any further help please call in to see us again.

Yours sincerely

John Salisbury
Operational Locality Manager